Defining the Historical, Physiological, Social and Environmental Factors of Diabetes Mellitus

Defining the Historical, Physiological, Social and Environmental Factors of Diabetes Mellitus

Austin Mardon
Avery Kemble
Gurleen Dhaliwal
Mehvish Masood
Adham H. El Sherbini
Varun Srikanth
Lydia C. Rehman
Harshita Saxena

Edited by Catherine Mardon

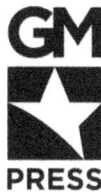

GM
★
PRESS

Cover Design & Typeset by Joshua Kramer

Print ISBN: 978-1-77369-828-1
eBook ISBN: 978-1-77369-829-8

Golden Meteorite Press
103 11919 82 St NW
Edmonton, AB T5B 2W3
www.goldenmeteoritepress.com

Contents

CHAPTER 1: THE MECHANISMS OF DIABETES
by Avery Kemble* HBHSc (c)

Introduction

Diabetes mellitus, or simply diabetes, is a group of metabolic disorders characterized by hyperglycemia (Schuster & Duvuuri, 2002). This hyperglycemia, also known as high blood sugar, is caused by deficiencies in insulin secretion, insulin action, or both (Schuster & Duvuuri, 2002). Insulin is a hormone that regulates blood sugar levels. Chronic hyperglycemia is associated with organ damage, especially in the eyes, kidneys, nerves, heart, and blood vessels, so management of blood sugar levels is critical (Schuster & Duvuuri, 2002).

Insulin

Insulin is an endocrine peptide hormone produced by the pancreas that regulates glycemia to maintain homeostasis, or ideal biological conditions (Petersen & Shulman, 2018). Glycemia refers to the amount of glucose in the blood, commonly called 'blood sugar level' (Health Canada, 2021). The biosynthesis of insulin begins with translating messenger RNA (mRNA) into preproinsulin, a polypeptide of 110 amino acids (Vasiljević et al., 2020). An mRNA is a form of genetic material formed from DNA through a process called transcription and then translated into proteins by the ribosomes inside the cell. Preproinsulin is like an immature form of insulin; it must undergo modifications to become the active hormone (Vasiljević et al., 2020).

There are four main parts to preproinsulin: a signal peptide sequence at the N-terminus end, then a B chain, which connects to a C-peptide, and an A chain at the C-terminus end (Vasiljević et al., 2020). The signal peptide sequence functions like a mailing address on an envelope (Choo et al., 2005); it directs the polypeptide to the endoplasmic reticulum (ER), which is an organelle inside the cell (Vasiljević et al., 2020). Inside the ER, the signal peptidase enzyme removes the signal peptide (Vasiljević et al., 2020). Enzymes called protein disulfide isomerases (PDIs) catalyze the formation of three disulfide bonds between cysteine residues (Vasiljević et al., 2020). Two of these bonds form bridges between the A-chain and B-chain, and one is within the A-chain itself (Vasiljević et al., 2020). This new polypeptide is called proinsulin. After the removal of the signal peptide and subsequent formation of the three disulfide bonds, proinsulin is transported through the Golgi body, another organelle inside the cell, to secretory granules (Vasiljević et al., 2020). Inside the secretory granules, two enzymes called proprotein convertase 1/3 (PC1/3) and carboxypeptidase E/H (CPE) further process the polypeptide, including completely cleaving the C-peptide, to form mature insulin (Vasiljević et al., 2020). A zinc (II) cation binds ionically to the Histidine (B10) residue to form the insulin hexamer (Vasiljević et al., 2020)

Insulin binds to receptors in the cell membrane to coordinate an anabolic response to glucose in the blood, where glucose is either oxidized or metabolized into glycogen (Petersen & Shulman, 2018). Glucose oxidation, formally known as glycolysis, converts glucose into a pyruvate molecule, which is used to create energy through cellular respiration (Petersen & Shulman, 2018). Glycogen is the storage form of glucose (Petersen & Shulman, 2018). It is a branched polymer comprised of linked glucose molecules (Adeva-Andany et al., 2016). It is stored primarily in the liver and skeletal muscle and can be broken down into glucose for cellular respiration as needed (Adeva-Andany et al., 2016).

Two signalling cascades allow insulin to maintain glucose homeostasis: insulin-mediated glucose uptake (IMGU) and glucose-stimulated insulin secretion (GSIS) (Vargas et al., 2021). Through the IMGU cascade, insulin lowers blood sugar levels (Vargas et al., 2021). The presence of insulin triggers the uptake of glucose by skeletal muscle and adipose tissue, where glucose gets metabolized into glycogen for storage (Vargas et al., 2021). The IMGU pathway also suppresses glucose generation in the liver to avoid further increasing blood sugar levels (Vargas et al., 2021). GSIS describes how the presence of glucose encourages the production of insulin.

Types of Diabetes

There are many different types of diabetes, the two most common being type 1 diabetes mellitus (T1DM) and type 2 diabetes mellitus (T2DM) (Canadian Diabetes Association, 2022). T1DM develops in childhood, while T2DM develops in adulthood due to a combination of external and biological factors (Centers for Disease Control and Prevention, 2021). While the specific biological and environmental factors differ in T1DM and T2DM, both involve an inherited predisposition to the disease, with the onset triggered by an environmental factor (American Diabetes Association, 2022).

Type 1 Diabetes

T1DM is an autoimmune condition where the destruction of the pancreatic β-cells leads to lifelong insulin deficiency and hyperglycemia (Weisman et al., 2020). 5-10% of individuals with diabetes have type 1 (Banday et al., 2020). It is also called insulin-dependent diabetes because individuals rely on alternative forms of insulin to regulate their blood sugar levels (Canadian Diabetes Association, 2022). Other names T1DM may be known as include juvenile-onset diabetes, ketosis-prone diabetes, and brittle diabetes of youth (Schuster & Duvuuri, 2002). The prevalence of T1DM is increasing worldwide by around 2-5% annually (Sapra & Bhandari, 2021).

While genetics play a significant role in the development of T1DM, external factors like diet or infection ultimately trigger its onset (Dean & McEntyre, 2004). In fact, the risk of T1DM for a monozygotic (identical) twin of someone with the disease is only 30%, indicating that biology is not the only factor (Schuster & Duvuuri, 2002). There has not yet been the discovery of one gene that causes T1DM. However, one locus on the short arm of chromosome 6 in the HLA class II region provides 40-50% of the inheritable diabetic risk (Schuster & Duvuuri, 2002). Viruses involved in the destruction of β-cells that can therefore trigger the onset of T1DM include coxsackie B, mumps, and cytomegalovirus (Schuster & Duvuuri, 2002).

The onset of T1DM typically occurs before adulthood but can occur at any age (Centers for Disease Control and Prevention, 2021). Approximately 45% of cases present before age 10, with onset peaking during ages four to six and 10 to 14 (Sapra & Bhandari, 2021). More than 85% of individuals with T1DM lack a family history of the disease (Sapra & Bhandari, 2021). Other autoimmune conditions have been associated with T1DM, including Grave's disease, vitiligo, and celiac disease (Schuster & Duvuuri, 2002). T1DM is diagnosed by testing blood glucose levels, often after a period of fasting (Sapra & Bhandari, 2021). Before onset, T1DM can be predicted by a test that looks for the presence of islet cell autoantibodies in the blood (Jia et al., 2020). An undiagnosed patient often presents with polyuria (frequent urination), polydipsia (excessive thirst), weight loss, and a fruity scent in their breath (Sapra & Bhandari, 2021). As type 1 diabetics cannot produce their own insulin, hormone treatments must be administered regularly (Sapra & Bhandari, 2021). This is done either through daily injections or by a machine known as an insulin pump.

Type 2 Diabetes

Type 2 diabetes mellitus is a chronic metabolic disease that typically onsets during adulthood (O'Reilly et al., 2011). It accounts for 90-95% of all diabetes cases and has been called non-insulin-dependent diabetes and adult-onset diabetes (American Diabetes Association, 2014). It is characterized by abnormalities in both insulin secretion and action (Brown et al., 2015). Unlike T1DM, the autoimmune destruction of β-cells does not occur, and individuals still tend to produce insulin (American Diabetes Association, 2014). As a result, patients do not often require insulin injections to survive (American Diabetes Association, 2014). The prevalence of T2DM in Canada has nearly doubled since 2000 and is a cause for concern (Brown et al., 2015). This form of diabetes has many possible complications and is the leading cause of blindness, end-stage renal disease, and non-traumatic amputation among Canadian adults (Brown et al., 2015). It is the seventh leading cause of death in Canada, with approximately two-thirds of the deaths due to heart disease or stroke (Brown et al., 2015). Biology plays a more significant role in the development of type 2 diabetes than type 1 (American Diabetes Association, 2022). However, most patients with T2DM are obese (American Diabetes Association, 2014), and weight management through healthy eating and exercising can significantly reduce one's risk (American Diabetes Association, 2022).

Gestational Diabetes

There are a few less common types of diabetes. Gestational diabetes mellitus (GDM) is a temporary form of diabetes that onsets during pregnancy, usually during the second or third trimester (Banday et al., 2020). It is different from pre-existing diabetes in pregnant patients as it typically resolves soon after childbirth or the termination of pregnancy (Banday et al., 2020). It occurs in 1-14% of all pregnancies, and the exact prevalence depends on the population under study (Banday et al., 2020). The rate is highest amongst people of Indian descent but is also high in pregnant people of Indigenous Australian, Middle Eastern, Filipina, Pacific Island, Mexican, and East Asian descent. The rate is lower amongst Black women and lowest amongst non-Hispanic white women. The risk of GDM increases with age, obesity, previous pregnancy with large babies, and a history of impaired glucose tolerance or gestational diabetes (Banday et al., 2020).

Individuals with gestational diabetes are usually asymptomatic, so diagnostic testing is standard for all pregnancies between 24 and 28 weeks (Centers for Disease Control and Prevention, 2021). During early pregnancy, blood glucose levels are usually below the normal range, but they increase during the third trimester (Banday et al., 2020). If they rise above a certain level, the patient is diagnosed with GDM.

Maturity-Onset Diabetes of the Young

Another form of diabetes is maturity-onset diabetes of the young (MODY): a heterogeneous disease in which most individuals are not insulin-dependent (Banday et al., 2020). MODY usually onsets before age 25 but is often misdiagnosed as type 1 or type 2 diabetes mellitus (Banday et al., 2020). MODY accounts for less than 2% of all diabetes cases and 1-6% of pediatric diabetes cases (Banday et al., 2020).

Several mutations can cause MODY. These mutations are in the specific genes involved in pancreatic β-cell function, which affect glucose sensing and subsequent insulin secretion (Banday et al., 2020). If the body cannot correctly determine its glycemic levels, it cannot secrete the correct amount of insulin to maintain homeostasis. Most individuals with MODY do not have defects in the action of insulin, meaning that the insulin they secrete does work properly (Banday et al., 2020). Researchers have identified 14 gene mutations that can lead to MODY (Banday et al., 2020). A patient will be diagnosed with a specific subtype of MODY depending on their genetic mutation (Banday et al., 2020). The two most common subtypes, MODY2 and MODY3, account for over 80% of all MODY cases (Banday et al., 2020). MODY1 and MODY5 account for 5% each, and the rarer subtypes account for the remaining cases (Banday et al., 2020). The mutations that cause MODY follows an autosomal dominant inheritance pattern, meaning only one parent must have a copy of the gene for it to affect the child (Banday et al., 2020). Because of this inheritance pattern, a child will only develop MODY if a parent has it.

Neonatal Diabetes

Neonatal diabetes mellitus (NDM), also called early-onset or congenital diabetes, is a rare form of diabetes mellitus diagnosed before six months of age (Banday et al., 2020). The global prevalence is only 1 per 500,000-300,000 live births (Banday et al., 2020). NDM is different from T1DM in that it is primarily of genetic origin (Banday et al., 2020). It can either be transient or permanent and is characterized by severe uncontrolled hyperglycemia along with hypoinsulinemia (insulin deficiency) (Banday et al., 2020). The genetic abnormalities lead to β-cell dysfunction and cell death (Banday et al., 2020). Individuals with NDM require insulin replacement therapy to survive (American Diabetes Association, 2014).

Transient neonatal diabetes mellitus, or TNDM, represents 55-60% of neonatal diabetes cases (Banday et al., 2020). It is often the result of a defect in ZAC/HYAMI imprinting (American Diabetes Association, 2014). Usually, TNDM resolves within 12-18 months after birth but comes back later in life as type 2 diabetes. Permanent neonatal diabetes mellitus (PNDM) is the rarer form of neonatal diabetes. It is typically caused by an autosomal dominant mutation in the ABCC8 and KCNJ11 genes (Banday et al., 2020). PNDM is also associated with syndromes such as immune-dysregulation, polyendocrinopathy, enteropathy, X-linked (IPEX) syndrome; and Wolcott-Rallison syndrome, the latter of which is the most common cause of PNDM (Banday et al., 2020). Unfortunately, it is not possible to predict whether neonatal diabetes will enter remission or remain permanent (Banday et al., 2020).

Conclusion

Diabetes mellitus is a diverse group of diseases, with varying causes and risk factors. Despite this heterogeneity, they are all characterized by persistent hyperglycemia and can result in a range of physiological complications. Diagnostic and therapeutic tools have improved significantly with the development of new technology and are continuing to improve quickly. However, diabetes can still result in deadly complications, so early diagnosis and management are crucial.

REFERENCES

Adeva-Andany, M. M., González-Lucán, M., Donapetry-García, C., Fernández-Fernández, C., & Ameneiros-Rodríguez, E. (2016). Glycogen metabolism in humans. *BBA Clinical, 5,* 85–100. https://doi.org/10.1016/J.BBACLI.2016.02.001

American Diabetes Association. (2014). Diagnosis and Classification of Diabetes Mellitus. *Diabetes Care, 37*(Supplement_1), S81–S90. https://doi.org/10.2337/DC14-S081

American Diabetes Association. (2022). *Learn the Genetics of Diabetes.* American Diabetes Association. https://www.diabetes.org/diabetes/genetics-diabetes

Banday, M. Z., Sameer, A. S., & Nissar, S. (2020). Pathophysiology of diabetes: An overview. *Avicenna Journal of Medicine, 10*(4), 174. https://doi.org/10.4103/AJM.AJM_53_20

Brown, K., Nevitte, A., Szeto, B., & Nandi, A. (2015). Growing social inequality in the prevalence of type 2 diabetes in Canada, 2004–2012. *Canadian Journal of Public Health, 106*(3), e132–e139. https://doi.org/10.17269/CJPH.106.4769

Canadian Diabetes Association. (2022). *What is diabetes?* Diabetes Canada. https://www.diabetes.ca/about-diabetes/what-is-diabetes

Centers for Disease Control and Prevention. (2021, April 27). *Diabetes Symptoms.* U.S. Department of Health & Human Services. https://www.cdc.gov/diabetes/basics/symptoms.html

Choo, K. H., Tan, T. W., & Ranganathan, S. (2005). SPdb - A signal peptide database. *BMC Bioinformatics, 6*(1), 1–8. https://doi.org/10.1186/1471-2105-6-249

Dean, L., & McEntyre, J. (2004). *The Genetic Landscape of Diabetes.* National Center for Biotechnology Information (US). https://www.ncbi.nlm.nih.gov/books/NBK1667/

Health Canada. (2021, December 13). *Diabetes in Canada in review, 2021.* Government of Canada. https://www.canada.ca/en/public-health/services/publications/diseases-conditions/diabetes-canada-review-2021.html

Jia, X., Gu, Y., High, H., & Yu, L. (2020). Islet autoantibodies in disease prediction and pathogenesis. *Diabetology International, 11*(1), 6. https://doi.org/10.1007/S13340-019-00414-9

O'Reilly, D. J., Xie, F., Pullenayegum, E., Gerstein, H. C., Greb, J., Blackhouse, G. K., Tarride, J. E., Bowen, J., & Goeree, R. A. (2011). Estimation of the impact of diabetes-related complications on health utilities for patients with type 2 diabetes in Ontario, Canada. *Quality of Life Research, 20*(6), 939–943. https://doi.org/10.1007/s11136-010-9828-9

Petersen, M. C., & Shulman, G. I. (2018). Mechanisms of Insulin Action and Insulin Resistance. *Physiological Reviews, 98*(4), 2133–2223. https://doi.org/10.1152/physrev.00063.2017

Sapra, A., & Bhandari, P. (2021). Diabetes Mellitus. *StatPearls.* https://www.ncbi.nlm.nih.gov/books/NBK551501/

Schuster, D. P., & Duvuuri, V. (2002). Diabetes mellitus. *Clinics in Podiatric Medicine and Surgery, 19*(1), 79–107. https://doi.org/10.1016/S0891-8422(03)00082-X

Vargas, E., Joy, N. v., & Sepulveda, M. A. C. (2021). Biochemistry, Insulin Metabolic Effects. *StatPearls.* https://www.ncbi.nlm.nih.gov/books/NBK525983/

Vasiljević, J., Torkko, J. M., Knoch, K. P., & Solimena, M. (2020). The making of insulin in health and disease. *Diabetologia, 63*(10), 1981–1989. https://doi.org/10.1007/s00125-020-05192-7

Weisman, A., Tu, K., Young, J., Kumar, M., Austin, P. C., Jaakkimainen, L., Lipscombe, L., Aronson, R., & Booth, G. L. (2020). Validation of a type 1 diabetes algorithm using electronic medical records and administrative healthcare data to study the population incidence and prevalence of type 1 diabetes in Ontario, Canada. *BMJ Open Diabetes Research and Care, 8*(1). https://doi.org/10.1136/bmjdrc-2020-001224

CHAPTER 2: DIABETES - THE ROAD TO DISCOVERY
by Gurleen Dhaliwal*, HBSc (c)

Introduction

Diabetes mellitus, commonly known as "diabetes," is one of the most complex chronic diseases studied and has an incredibly long road to discovery. In fact, one might say that this road is still ongoing and bustling with breakthroughs. Through this chapter, we explore the milestones of scientific discovery beginning from as early as 1500 BC up to the present. By understanding the history of scientific discovery and beliefs, we see how significant advancements can benefit societies. Not only is it interesting to learn about how current treatments and knowledge came to be, but how thinking and understanding are altered. Centuries of negated hypotheses and proposed truths led to now, so let us delve deep into the past of diabetes.

Ancient Centuries at a Glance

Diabetes has intriguing Egyptian, Indian and Chinese traces discovered in ancient medical books. In Ebers Papyrus, an Egyptian medical text dating back to 1500 BC, passages were discovered with a possible connection to diabetes (Karamanou et al., 2016). They described patients experiencing frequent thirst and excessive urination who were treated with plant extracts (Karamanou et al., 2016). These plant extract treatments consisted of decoctions of grain, bones, green lead, earth, grit, and wheat (Vecchio et al., 2018). That being said, historians and translators of the Ebers Papyrus, such as Paul Ghalioungui, argued that the description is a poor and inadequate representation of diabetes (Karamanou et al., 2016). Another book of ancient Egyptian texts called the Kahun Papyrus

(2000 BC) had a chapter titled "Treatment of a thirsty woman." The text, unfortunately, was missing and speculated to contain a recipe for diabetes treatment (Karamanou et al., 2016).

Interestingly, around 500 BC, diabetes was referred to as "madhumeha" in Samhita by Sushruta, a famous Indian physician (Karamanou et al., 2016, Vecchio et al., 2018). The term "madhumeha" meant honey-like urine, which pointed out the sticky sensation and the sweet smell of urine that attracted ants (Karamanou et al., 2016). The surgeon additionally noted how the disease seemed to impact the rich castes and had a connection with unrestrained food consumption, including cereals, sweets, and rice (Karamanou et al., 2016).

The first case where symptoms of diabetes were categorized under a singular specific disease occurred in ancient China (Karamanou et al., 2016). Zhang Zhongjing, an individual who was believed to be the Chinese Hippocrates, described polydipsia (excessive thirst), polyuria (excessive urination), and loss of weight as symptoms of a particular disease (Karamanou et al., 2016). Independently, Chen Chuan was a 7th century AD Chinese physician who named diabetes Hsiao kho ping, His colleague had diabetes, and Chuan proposed a treatment in the form of abstinence from wine, salt, and sex (Karamanou et al., 2016).

As the 8th century progressed, it was noted that diabetic patients frequently developed skin infections (Karamanou et al., 2016). In the 11th century, an Arabo-Islamic physician Avicenna observed diabetic complications, which included gangrene and sexual dysfunction (Karamanou et al., 2016). Years later, the philosopher Moises Maimonides rose to relevance and explained diabetes in detail. In his description, he included the symptoms of acidosis, a condition of excessive acid accumulation in the body (Karamanou et al., 2016).

Although these pieces of knowledge were informative, the advancements were relatively vague and unsatisfactory descriptions of diabetes mellitus. The first accurate account of the disease, its symptoms, and its complexities was by Aretaeus of Cappadocia in the second century (Karamanou et al., 2016).

The Origin of the Term 'Diabetes Mellitus'

Aretaeus was a Greco-Roman physician in the second century. Before Aretaeus, Claudius Galenus, commonly referred to as Galen, and other medical authors mentioned the common symptoms of diabetes, which included thirst, polyuria, and the possibility of death (Karamanou et al., 2016). Galen initially used the term diarrhea urinoma (diarrhea of the urine), and Arataeus later introduced the term 'diabetes' (Karamanou et al., 2016, Vecchio et al., 2018). Diabetes comes from the Greek word "διαβήτης" (diabaino), which translates to 'the fluid that passes through' (Karamanou et al., 2016, Laios et al., 2012). Aretaeus' precise observation of diabetes was authentic and detailed, which is quite impressive as the disease remained rare during that time (Karamanou et al., 2016). His clinical presentation, as well as simplification of the disease, is remembered for its accuracy. A translation of Arataeus' works by Francis Adams (1856) mentions an apposite quotation of Arataeus' from a passage that reads the following:

"Diabetes is a remarkable affliction, not very frequent among men... The course is the common one, namely, the kidneys and the bladder; for the patients never stop making water, but the flow is incessant, as if from the opening of aqueducts. The nature of the disease, then, is chronic, and it takes a long period to form; but the patient is short-lived, if the constitution of the disease be completely established; for the melting is rapid, the death speedy...Hence, the disease appears to me to have got

the name diabetes as if from the Greek word διαβήτης (which signifies a siphon), because the fluid does not remain in the body, but uses the man's body as a ladder, whereby to leave it. They survive not for long, for they pass urine with pain, and the emaciation is dreadful; nor does any great portion of the drink get into the system, and many parts of the flesh pass out along with the urine" (p. 398-399).

In the 17th century, English physician and anatomist Thomas Willis wrote a chapter about the "pissing evil" (Karamanou et al., 2016, Vecchio et al., 2018). He mentioned the sweetness of urine, which became a rediscovery since Willis was unaware of Sushrata's early discovery (Karamanou et al., 2016). From this, the term "mellitus" came to be, the Latin word for sweet.

Thomas Willis, Matthew Dobson, and Claude Bernard

Thomas Willis believed diabetes was not due to the kidneys but due to an infection of the blood (Karamanou et al., 2016). He stated that eating habits, as well as psychological statuses, such as sadness or prolonged grief, played a role in the disease. Willis additionally exemplified the case of a noble earl who began to "excessively piss...and void almost a gallon and a half of limpid, clear, and wonderful sweet water, that tasted as if it has been mixed with honey" (Karamanou et al., 2016). He suggested treatments of thick and cool diets, including starch, slimy vegetables, and rice, which helped patients improve. The physician could not discover why the urine was sweet (Karamanou et al., 2016). However, this particular discovery was propelled by English physician Matthew Dobson about a century later when he noted the presence of sugar in the urine. Dobson experimented with the liquid by boiling urine to dryness and discovering a crystalline leftover with the taste of brown sugar (Karamanou et al., 2016). After discovering that an excess of sugar was the cause of the sweetness, he published it in "Medical Observations and Enquiries" (Vecchio et al., 2018).

Likewise, another key figure in the 19th century on the road to discovering diabetes is Claude Bernard (Karamanou et al., 2016). He was a French physiologist who initially was a playwright with a passion for theatre before he delved into medicine. Bernard's contributions played a significant role in the studies of metabolism and diabetes. He tested a hypothesis regarding the role of the pancreas in diabetes (Karamanou et al., 2016). In his experiments, he ruled out the lungs as a cause of diabetes and demonstrated that sugar is present in animal blood without a food supply. Bernard analyzed the liver tissues of dogs in an experimental group fed carbohydrate diets, and dogs in a control group fed only meat (Karamanou et al., 2016). He discovered that a large amount of glucose was missing from other organs and deduced that the liver stored a starchy substance, which he later called glycogen, that was turned into glucose and discharged into the blood. Bernard believed an excess of glycogen release was the cause of diabetes (Karamanou et al., 2016).

The Discovery of Insulin

During the pre-insulin era, treatments to control diabetes were largely diet-intensive and pharmacological (Vecchio et al., 2018). Diabetic patients were suggested to compensate for any metabolic decrease with hyper-caloric diets (Vecchio et al., 2018). However, it was observed that reducing calorie consumption improved diabetic symptoms and, consequently, the diet became restricted (Vecchio et al., 2018). Over the next few years, sugar-free and low-calorie diets rose to popularity until the final discovery of insulin.

In 1889, Oskar Minkowski and Joseph von Mering experimented on dogs and learned that removing the pancreas resulted in diabetes (Lakhtakia,

2013). This crucial discovery led to a renewed focus on the pancreas gland and was necessary for what was to come. Paul Langherans discovered the 'islets of Langherans' in 1869, which are groups of cells spread across the pancreas (Lakhtakia 2013). Decades later, by 1916, Sir Edward Albert Sharpey-Schafer identified that these pancreatic islets secreted a substance that could lower blood glucose levels (Lakhtakia, 2013, Vecchio et al., 2018). He termed the substance "insulin" with reference to the Latin word "insula" which meant island (Lakhtakia, 2013, Vecchio et al., 2018).

Frederick Banting and John MacLeod were both influenced by the recent advancements and unlearned aspects of the pancreas' role in diabetes. For one, it was not known how the organ impacts sugar production and usage (Karamanou et al., 2016). It was assumed by the 19th century that the pancreas secretes a hormone into the blood that spreads to the tissues, allowing them to use the glucose or pass it to the liver for storage (Karamanou et al., 2016).

Banting worked with a medical student, Charles Best, at the University of Toronto, where they both experimented on dogs. In these studies, they degenerated, removed, and purified an extract of the Langerhans islands (Karamanou et al., 2016, Vecchio et al., 2018). The prime struggle was to separate this extract from the pancreatic exocrine tissue (Vecchio et al., 2018). Banting and Best then injected the extract into the dogs and observed a considerable drop in blood sugar (Karamanou et al., 2016). Chemist James Collip joined Banting and Best and helped improve their extraction and purification method (Karamanou et al., 2016). This extract was the first substance that could regulate glucose in an animal with diabetes. They had achieved their goal to remove and isolate the secreted substance from the pancreatic islets known now as insulin.

The substance previously named "insletin" was changed to "insulin" by Macleod (Karamanou et al., 2016). The following phase was human-testing. On January 11, 1922, Leonard Thompson, a 14-year-old diabetic patient, was the first patient to be injected with insulin at Toronto General Hospital (Karamanou et al., 2016, Vecchio et al., 2018). During the 19th and 20th centuries, eating as little as possible was a dietary treatment for the disease that physicians still upheld (Karamanou et al., 2016). However, after being administered 15 mL of insulin, the boy's condition worsened (Karamanou et al., 2016, Vecchio et al., 2018). On January 23, an improved form of insulin, thanks to Collip, was administered to Thompson, leading to very successful results (Karamanou et al., 2016). His blood glucose levels dropped drastically, and any urinary ketones went away. Insulin became a considerable success and lifesaver, and in 1923, it became a product accessible to the public (Karamanou et al., 2016). This sensational and revolutionary discovery won Banting and MacLeod the Nobel Prize for the discovery of insulin. Banting shared his award with Best, and MacLeod shared his award with Collip, both of whom were excluded (Karamanou et al., 2016).

Sir Harold Himsworth

The discovery of insulin was very relevant to both types of diabetes; however, when were the two main types differentiated? Type 1 diabetes is characterized as insulin-dependent, whereas type 2 diabetes is known as non-insulin-dependent (Karamanou et al., 2016). One of the earliest pieces of research portraying a distinction between the two types was by Sir Harold Himsworth. Himsworth, in his 1936 Lancet paper, wrote that diabetes could be differentiated into two types: insulin-sensitive and insulin-insensitive. This prompted him to believe that a different type of diabetes mellitus was not due to a lack of insulin but insensitivity to insulin (Himsworth, 1936). Himsworth could not test and compare the blood glucose levels of diabetic patients following insulin administration because every patient is unique (Himsworth, 1936). Thus, he sought to test an animal's sensitivity to insulin through a new method. He stated in his article that "if glucose and insulin are given simultaneously to a normal animal, then the extent to which the injected insulin suppresses the hyperglycemia, consequent upon the administration of glucose, is determined by the sensitivity of the animal to insulin" (Himsworth, 1936). After conducting this test, it led to two results. In patient I, the injection of insulin had little to no consequence on the hyperglycaemic symptoms (Himsworth, 1936). Contrastingly, in patient II, the hyperglycemia subdued, and there was a drop in blood glucose as well (Himsworth, 1936). Himsworth concluded that patient I was insulin-insensitive and patient II was insulin-sensitive (Himsworth, 1936). Today, 'sensitive' and 'insensitive' are commonly referred to as 'type 1' diabetes and 'type 2' diabetes. Sir Harold Himsworth's research was pioneering and paved the way toward additional advancements in knowledge and treatment of diabetes mellitus.

Conclusion

Throughout the centuries, the symptoms and causes of diabetes mellitus have been examined and observed. Groundbreaking scientific discovery has led us to modern day treatments and understandings of diabetes. Following the discovery of insulin, many additional advancements led to findings on the structure of insulin, proinsulin, and pancreas transplantation. Techniques have been improved to purify and prepare insulin. Additionally, more products have been released to the market, making the management of diabetes easier for individuals living with chronic disease. Several promising biomedical and scientific approaches are continuously being discovered, and research in understanding diabetes is advancing. The road to discovery holds a future of milestones to come.

REFERENCES

Adams, F. (1856). The extant works of Aretaeus, the Cappadocian. London: Sydenham Society.

Himsworth, H. P. (1936). Diabetes Mellitus: Its Differentiation Into Insulin-Sensitive And Insulin-Insensitive Types. *The Lancet, 227*(5864), 127-130. https://doi.org/10.1016/S0140-6736(01)36134-2.

Karamanou, M., Protogerou, A., Tsoucalas, G., Androutsos, G., Poulakou-Rebelakou, E. (2016). Milestones in the history of diabetes mellitus: The main contributors. *World Journal of Diabetes, 7*(1), 1-7. https://doi.org/10.4239%2Fwjd.v7.i1.1.

Laios, K., Karamanou, M., Saridaki, Z., Androutsos, G. (2012). Arataeus of Cappadocia and the first description of diabetes. *Hormones, 11*(1), 109-113. https://doi.org/10.1007/BF03401545.

Lakhtakia, R. (2013). The History of Diabetes Mellitus. *Sultan Qaboos University Medical Journal, 13*(3), 368-370. https://doi.org/10.12816%2F0003257.

Vecchio, I., Tornali, C., Bragazzi, N. L., Martini, M. (2018). The Discovery of Insulin: An Important Milestone in the History of Medicine. *Frontiers in Endocrinology, 9,* 613. https://doi.org/10.3389/fendo.2018.00613.

CHAPTER 3: MANAGEMENT OF DIABETES - TECHNOLOGIES, MEDICATIONS, PREVENTION
by Mehvish Masood*, HBMSc (c)

As previously implied, diabetes is a complex and multifaceted disease that impacts the lives of those diagnosed with it in complex ways. Fortunately, our increased understanding and research into diabetes has dramatically increased our ability to find ways to manage this condition. New technologies regarding diabetes management have allowed individuals, who previously had short life spans, to live long and happy lives. As research has become more advanced, we have developed many forms and ways to manage diabetes. Each one has different benefits and efficiencies that are important to know. Consequently, this chapter will discuss different aspects of diabetes management, which include technologies, medications, and prevention.

Therapeutic Medications

Many forms of therapeutic medications can be used to help diabetic patients. The use of each type depends on the type of diabetes the individual has and the lifestyle that the individual leads. It is recommended that those with diabetes should consult with their doctor before pursuing any lines of treatment in terms of therapeutic medications.

Insulin therapy is one of the most commonly known treatment medications for diabetes. Since its discovery by Fredrick Banting, its commercial use has progressed and developed (Hu & Jia, 2019). Generally speaking, patients with type 1 diabetes are insulin-dependent, which is not necessarily the case for patients with type 2 diabetes. In the latter case, lifestyle modifications and other therapeutic medications tend to be used first before insulin is used as a course of action. In terms of development, there are three types of insulin preparations that depend on the production techniques: human insulin, animal insulin, and insulin analogues. Insulin preparations are further divided into various categories depending on their role of action. For example, there are rapid-acting insulins, long-acting insulins, and premixed insulins. Notably, unlike other therapeutic medications, insulin requires more healthcare oversight and patient self-monitoring skills to be used efficiently (Hu & Jia, 2019).

Outside of insulin, metformin can be used as a therapeutic medication to treat diabetes. Generally used for type 2 diabetes patients, this medication is considered the first line of treatment, especially with obese patients. Currently, metformin's mechanism of action is not fully understood by researchers. Traditionally, this medication is thought to increase glucose sensitivity in the liver by decreasing the amount of glucose made by the same organ (Hu & Jia, 2019). However, there is increasing evidence that suggests that metformin impacts glucose production and changes within the gut. Nonetheless, metformin has shown to be extremely beneficial for T2DM in many ways. This medication has significantly reduced the mortality of type 2 diabetes-related deaths and other side effects. It has also been shown to help lower the weight of patients. That being said, adverse reactions to this medication tend to occur within organs of the digestive system (Hu & Jia, 2019).

Another therapeutic medication for type 2 diabetes is sulfonylureas. These medications are insulin secretagogues, which are substances that cause another substance to be secreted. Insulin is secreted through a complicated mechanism, involving potassium and calcium channels, among other components (Hu & Jia, 2019). For the most part, sulfonylurea drugs are categorized as first and second-generation agents. First-generation drugs have weaker effects, shorter action durations, and more adverse reactions when compared to second-generation drugs. Hypoglycemia, as in low blood sugar, is the most common adverse reaction to sulfonylureas and is commonly observed in patients that are taking long-acting sulfonylurea agents (Hu & Jia, 2019).

Thiazolidinediones (TZD) are therapeutic agents that work differently than sulfonylureas. TZDs mechanism of action involves increasing insulin sensitivity, especially in the peripheral tissues, by activating a special factor in the nucleus. Furthermore, they promote the breakdown of glucose through a metabolic process called oxidation (Hu & Jia, 2019). Alternatively, TZDs increase the synthesis of glycogen, a storage molecule for glucose, and decrease the creation of glucose in the liver. In addition to all the different mechanisms listed, there are even more ways that TZDs work to aid patients with type 2 diabetes. Much research is being put into understanding these mechanisms and potential side effects of TZDs (Hu & Jia, 2019).

Another therapeutic medication is SGLT2 inhibitors. Diabetes is often damaging to the body because of hyperglycemia, as in high blood sugar levels. SGLT2 inhibitors work by increasing the glucose excretion from the kidney. The kidney is the site of excretion for many different substances. Generally speaking, the kidney does not excrete glucose because the body wants to conserve it. For this reason, SGLT2 reabsorbs most of the glucose back into the body to prevent its secretion. These drugs stop SGLT2 glucose channels from reabsorbing glucose, decreasing a patient's hyperglycemia. Additionally, when compared to non-diabetic patients, SGLT2 channels are overexpressed in diabetic patients' kidneys(Hu & Jia, 2019).Therefore, the overall effect of SGLT2 drugs is hypoglycemia, and low blood sugar levels. SGLT2 inhibitors also cause other effects in the body. For example, it can increase blood plasma glucagon levels and improve insulin resistance. Clinical trials have demonstrated that SGLT2 inhibitors can significantly improve blood glucose, reduce weight, and control blood pressure. With that being said, SGLT2 inhibitors also have several adverse side effects. Generally speaking, urinary tract infections and genital infections are the most common effects. However, some rare adverse effects include ketoacidosis, orthostatic hypotension, postural dizziness, and increased urinary calcium excretion. Nonetheless, SGLT2 is well tolerated in most research (Hu & Jia, 2019).

Overall, therapeutic medications are useful in managing diabetes. Whether it be through insulin, TZDs, or metformin, all the different medications have helped diabetic patients manage their condition. With that being said, some drawbacks to therapeutic medications, including adverse side effects in patients, must be considered.Regardless, therapeutic medications are a productive first step in tackling diabetes and should be seriously considered an essential form of management for diabetes.

Technologies

In addition to therapeutic medications, there are other ways diabetes can be managed. One of such avenues includes technology. The technology works differently from therapeutic medications because it provides aid for both motivational and educational support. Education comes in the form of letting patients learn routines related to diabetes management and new practices. On the other hand, daily support for diabetes can aid with healthy eating, taking medication, blood glucose monitoring, and more. This section will discuss these different technologies, as well as the potential benefits and drawbacks that are associated with them.

Mobile health applications can be a helpful technological aid in diabetes self-management. This form of technology is beneficial for several reasons. Firstly, it is an accessible form of technology that can overcome barriers to provider access. With the inability of many individuals to access healthcare providers, this form of technology is beneficial. Alternatively, mobile phones allow the ability to communicate and process data in real-time (Hunt, 2015). This multifaceted aspect of mobile phones increases the convenience for users and comes in many forms. As in, users can access graphs that monitor changes in blood glucose, direct communication with healthcare providers in real-time, and receive reminders about self-management. This could help, for example, by letting participants see how changes in diet and exercise benefits participants. However, there are some drawbacks to this form of technology. For example, individuals that struggle with understanding how mobile phones work could struggle with these features (Hunt, 2015).

Another form of technology that is highly beneficial for diabetes is internet-based interventions. This is highly advantageous because of its ease of access around the world and can help give support, motivation, and education for self-management behaviours. Internet-based interventions are multifaceted in providing different information forms for education, patient feedback, behaviour tracking, and more. Different studies have suggested that internet-based interventions are highly effective in increasing the self-management of diabetes (Hunt, 2015).

Technology has shown to be a highly effective way to manage diabetes. Whether in the form of mobile health applications or internet-based interventions, these highly complex and multifaceted forms of aid are making the lives of those using these technologies much better.

Prevention of Type 2 Diabetes

Another element of diabetes management involves prevention. This element involves decreasing the likelihood of having diabetes and mitigating risk factors of diabetes through lifestyle modifications. With the healthcare system slowly being overburdened by the increasing rise in the cases of diabetes, implementing such preventions will be an essential part of mitigating diabetes. With that being said, there are two types of risk factors for diabetes. The first main risk factor is genetics, an element that cannot be consciously controlled. The other risk factors are related to lifestyle, which primarily involves dietary components, sedentary lifestyles, and being overweight (Hussain et al., 2007). All of these elements will be discussed.

As mentioned previously, being overweight is a risk factor for diabetes. There has been a correlation between the rise of obesity and the cases of diabetes. The exact mechanism between these two elements has yet to be established, but there are theories regarding various biological elements that are thought to be associated with diabetes (Hussain et al., 2007). Another risk factor involves dietary concerns and food habits. Weight gain and obesity are associated with an increased risk for diabetes. With diet being correlated to weight gain, it is important to discuss the impact of one's diet on diabetes. Generally speaking, low-fat diets prevent type 2 diabetes, and high monounsaturated fat intake can improve glycemic control (Hussain et al., 2007). Alternatively, a sedentary lifestyle is a risk factor for diabetes. Independent of body size, inactivity has been identified as a risk factor. Exercise or regular physical activity is associated with beneficial effects for diabetes prevention (Hussain et al., 2007).

There are different forms of prevention strategies that can be used to mitigate the risk factors. They are categorized according to their targets and ability to make a change. The three categories of primary prevention are downstream, midstream, and upstream prevention. Programs that target the most high-risk individuals are downstream prevention strategies. Midstream prevention programs target those believed to have an increased risk for diabetes. Alternatively, programs that target entire populations through, for example, public policy and environmental interventions are considered upstream prevention programs (Hussain et al., 2007). Generally speaking, upstream programs have the greatest potential for diabetes prevention but are very logistically complex to implement. Regardless, school children, young individuals, specific ethnic groups, and women with gestational diabetes can be some target groups for prevention strategies. Notably, increased physical activity and decreased consumption of energy-based foods is the best strategy for diabetes prevention (Hussain et al., 2007). Implementing these changes would require the efforts of those in government, policy change, and much more. The hope is that societies in the future will move in this direction to decrease the incidents of diabetes.

Conclusion

Diabetes management is a complex disease that requires many different components to consider. For example, it can involve therapeutic medications, which have benefits and possible side effects. Management also involves implementing technology that can help in self-management and education. Alternatively, prevention strategies targeting different populations to mitigate risk factors can be used for diabetes management. As a whole, diabetes is a complex disease. For this reason, it is important to seriously consider how all these elements play a role in helping those with the disease and work at making them all accessible and efficient to those needing them. If we can do so, we will have helped those with diabetes have much better, stronger, and happier lives.

REFERENCES

Hu, C., & Jia, W. (2019). Therapeutic medications against diabetes: What we have and what we expect. *Advanced drug delivery reviews, 139*, 3–15. https://doi.org/10.1016/j.addr.2018.11.008

Hunt CW. Technology and diabetes self-management: An integrative review. *World J Diabetes. 2015;6*(2):225-233. doi:10.4239/wjd.v6.i2.225

Hussain, A., Claussen, B., Ramachandran, A., & Williams, R. (2007). Prevention of type 2 diabetes: a review. *Diabetes research and clinical practice, 76*(3), 317–326. https://doi.org/10.1016/j.diabres.2006.09.0

CHAPTER 4: GLOBAL PERSPECTIVES ON DIABETES HEALTH DISPARITIES

by Adham El Sherbini*

Diabetes and Social Determinants of Health

The social determinants of health (SDH), defined by the World Health Organization (WHO) as the non-medical causes of diseases, are based upon the socio-economic factors and environmental conditions that shape an individual's life and the outcomes of a chronic condition (CMHA, 2022). The SDH has shaped the way healthcare practitioners, policymakers, and researchers think of disease. Comparatively, the socio-economic factors can be far more influential on the health outcomes of a disease rather than just the medical effects of the disease itself (Bernazzani, 2016). In a progressive world that is focused on solutions to disease management, understanding and implementing SDHs as a means of understanding the burden of disease is critical to reducing poor health outcomes, hospitalization, and overall economic cost (Islam, 2019). As thousands of epidemiologists and public health scientists globally work better to understand the impact of SDHs on specific conditions, its application in the hospital setting requires a deep understanding of implementation science, including qualitative and quantitative research.

As of 2019, approximately 463 million individuals have diabetes (T1DM and T2DM) globally, and this number is projected to increase to 700 million by 2045 (Saeedi et al., 2019). With half a billion individuals diagnosed with diabetes, it is necessary that this condition is critically evaluated. Both types of diabetes are highly manageable conditions with numerous non-genetic factors; thus, reducing the barriers to management is critical to avoid further implications. Understanding the dynamics of how social factors can impact diabetes can be a longitudinal step for healthcare practitioners in treating this disease.

Youth and Early Childhood Development

Type 2 Diabetes Mellitus (T2DM), understood as the misuse of glucose by the body has been typically associated with those above the age of 30 (Westman, 2021). However, this claim has been disproven as its proportionality continues to increase, alongside those with type 1 Diabetes Mellitus (T1DM) (National Center for Biotechnology Information, 2022). Specifically for those of more affected ethnicity, the prevalence of diabetes in younger adolescents continues to prevail (Spanakis & Golden, 2013). Although younger age is not necessarily a risk factor, many common social factors associated with this population serve as so. For one, children tend to be less understanding and aware of the consequences of unhealthy eating or an absence of exercise, both of which are severe risk factors for T2DM (New Research Uncovers Concerning Increases in Youth Living with Diabetes in the U.S., 2016). Other risk factors for a younger generation include high sugar diets, genetic diabetes, and the mental health implications that could translate into diabetes (Temneanu et al., 2016).

Racial Disparities in the Management of Diabetes

The current existing literature outlines the various associations between the prevalence and relationships between ethnicity and the onset of diabetes. Currently, in Canada, for individuals of South Asian ethnicities, the current incidence of diabetes is 3.4 times higher than in other ethnic populations (Ethnicity and Type 2 Diabetes, 2022). Research also suggests that this number may be upwards of six times higher than other ethnic populations (Narayan & Kanaya, 2020). Although geographical location and cultural practices can be associated with diabetes, the poor diabetes management in this community explains this significant number. Regarding cultural practices, many traditional diets consisted of higher sugar and salt content, leading to more insulin resistance (Muilwijk et al., 2018). The poor management of the condition is likely associated with barriers within healthcare, such as a lack of culturally inclusive treatment programs, absence of cultural training for medical providers, and the lack of respect for non-western methodologies (Chin et al., 2001). As healthcare works in a hierarchy where patients are expected to follow physician orders, health literacy becomes a sufficient barrier for many individuals. Additionally, this population group is also at high risk of developing other cardiovascular diseases (Patel et al., 2021). It is necessary to note that some research has found a genetic component for the South Asian community, such as a Nature study which concluded that six differing genes in this population were exceptionally subject to T2DM (Kooner et al., 2011). There also remains abdominal obesity, muscle metabolism, and fat metabolism factors, all of which are plausible associations with a spike in T2DM among the south Asian community (Pandit et al., 2012).

Other populations that face disproportionate rates of diabetes in Canada include Black (African, Caribbean) and Indigenous communities in North America. Black populations have double the occurrence of diabetes relative to their caucasian counterparts, and the African continent has the largest number of undiagnosed individuals with diabetes (Ethnicity and Type 2 Diabetes, 2022). As of 2021, the number of undiagnosed Africans has been reported to be as high as 13 million (Diabetes in Africa, 2022). A major component of this increased prevalence is the substantial racial discrimination this population faces. As a result of these racial injustices, African Americans have the highest number of undiagnosed T2DM in America, and self-reported racial discrimination was also associated with a reduction in quality of care and increased complications (Factors Contributing to Higher Incidence of Diabetes for Black Americans,

2018) (Peek et al., 2011). To add, the majority of self-reported racial discrimination in the case of diabetes was typically uninsured and low-income, culminating in a problematic public health issue. Racism is a social determinant of health that primarily affects communities of colour, and without proper intervention, it can hold life-altering complexities. To add, ensuring that healthcare practitioners are socially informed about the social determinants against racial groups is crucial, as they play a vital role in the health outcomes of diabetes for at-risk populations.

Similarly, there are a variety of reasons for how the complications of diabetes affect populations. For instance, the Native American population in the United States has a 45.3% chance of getting retinopathy as a complication of diabetes (Spanakis & Golden, 2013). Nephropathy, in both Native and African Americans, is the leading community for exhibiting microvascular complications as a complication. Thus, changing a system, where colonialism and racism create barriers for vulnerable minority populations can result in positive health outcomes and community empowerment.

Geographic Location

Geographic location has a great impact on the prevalence of diabetes, as there are various genetic, environmental, and socioeconomic conditions that predispose and increase the risk in certain populations (Bernazzani, 2016). For example, in the United States, fast-food chains, lack of walkability, and cultural acceptance of health-deterrent symptoms all lead to the nation being one of the leading locations of diabetes cases (Wu et al., 2014). These reasons continue to follow through when comparing urban and rural, as many urban locations contain far unhealthier diabetes management pillars. According to a published research paper, city corporations had the highest prevalence of diabetes, followed by small towns, and then rural areas in those above the age of 35 in Bangladesh

(Asaduzzaman et al., 2018). Although clear reasoning is yet to be defined, the abundance of unhealthy foods and lack of walkability within urban areas may explain such a high prevalence.

Gender

For nearly all medical conditions, research has been conducted to understand the difference in the sex outcomes regarding the disease. Although the male and female anatomy are different, there remain many social factors that can serve as SDHs inflicting on the prevalence of diabetes (Bates et al., 2009). Based on the CDC, although the male population is more likely to be diagnosed with diabetes, females are more susceptible to complications (CDC, 2022). Ignoring the biological factors, the difference in socioeconomic status (SES), otherwise understood as the combined social and economic measure of an individual, and psychosocial between the two sexes can explain the diabetes prevalence (Winkleby et al., 1992). A Canadian study found that among women over the age of 40 years, a generally low SES was associated with a higher prevalence of diabetes (Bird et al., 2015). Generally speaking, studies have found a more significant association between low SES and diabetes in women than men after controlling for risk factors, such as obesity and physical activity. However, it is important to note that a systematic review in the International Journal of Epidemiology concluded that both sexes are susceptible to T2DM when a low SES is in play (Tang et al., 2003). Although SES is a complicated and variable measure, its strong association with women can be understood. One study found that specific variables of a low SES, such as food insecurity or a lower income, were strong predictors of diabetes in women (Rivera et al., 2015). Additional factors are that women are more vulnerable to stress and deprivation of sleep; factors that are strongly tied in with low SES. In addition to the research on how diabetes impacts females and males, there is limited research in understanding gender diversity in diabetes health research. There should be an inclusion of understanding of the way diabetes impacts people of all gender identities, and how the health outcomes of diabetes are directly correlated to gender.

It is also important to critically appraise the trends amongst sex and the management of diabetes. For instance, evidence illustrates that men are more likely to be more physically active compared to women (Azevedo et al., 2007). However, despite this statistic, evidence shows that women typically have healthier diets than men, which consist of fruits and vegetables (Bärebring et al., 2020). Interestingly, another study found that the association between Body Mass Index (BMI), gender, and diabetes was more robust for men than women (Zhang et al., 2019). The relationship between diabetes and gender/sex is complicated, as there are many social and non-social factors involved in understanding the physiology and management of diabetes.

Income

The relationship between income and diabetes has been well established in the literature. For example, one Canadian study found that those in the lowest income bracket (<$15,000) had a 4.14 times higher chance of receiving diabetes than the highest income bracket (> $80,000) (Dinca-Panaitescu et al., 2011). This association is quite redundant amongst the literature and it explains previously mentioned research, such as a low SES correlating with diabetes. That is, income, alongside occupation, is the focal point of defining SES and therefore explains that relationship (Worthy et al., 2020). Moreover, low income makes it exceptionally difficult to eat a healthier diet, as processed foods are cheap. Additionally, a low income can often be related to psychological stress, which is also a factor in an increased prevalence of diabetes, especially among women (Jena et al., 2018).

Another Canadian study investigated the rate of rehospitalization of diabetes with respect to income (Gupta et al., 2020). They found that there is no association between income and rehospitalization for women who have a primary or secondary diagnosis of diabetes. However, men in the lowest household income bracket had a higher rate of rehospitalization when diabetes was a primary diagnosis or secondary diagnosis. The concept of income, while complex, is a social determinant of diabetes that can be managed. The association between low income, high prevalence of diabetes, and increased rehospitalization should be of concern to the government. Exploring solutions, such as Guaranteed Annual Income (GAI) or increasing wages to a living wage, could be possible economic solutions to mitigating the barriers to managing diabetes and further improving health outcomes.

Social Capital

Social capital is best defined as the relationships one has, better termed a "network" (Gannon & Roberts, 2018). Although very simple, it has been proven to be a large-scale factor in diseases and syndromes. For context, in a study done to understand how social capital in Japan impacts the health outcomes of diabetes, the researchers engaged in qualitative research by utilizing questionnaires titled "trust in people in the community", "social supports", and "social relationships" (Yamada et al., 2018). This same study found that social capital was a strong indicator of positive health outcomes associated with diabetes. Specifically, the study reported that specific factors, such as wishing to be helped negatively influence diabetes management, while other factors, such as "participation in favourite activity" bettered diabetes control. More importantly, the study concluded that social capital positively impacted diabetes and its management. The reason that the "hope to be helped" factor was negatively influential in the Japanese population was likely the level of dependency in the community. The Japanese are big on dependency and teamwork, making the self-management of diabetes quite difficult. This shows how even research studies have numerous social determinants of health that are nearly impossible to separate from one another. Another study focused on additional social capital characteristics and found that trust and solitary directly affected on diabetes (Moradi et al., 2017). That is, a lack of social trust affects diabetes. Therefore, researchers and public health scientists should focus on deriving all the social capital factors that influence diabetes. This guideline can be exceptionally effective in implementing ideas and solutions to reduce the general prevalence of diabetes within the community while providing a progressive population effectively managing the disease.

Conclusion

Public health research, interventions, and health promotion continue to become more advanced in highlighting the disease burden and socio-economic factors that impede health status. Advancing the field of public health to understand how the SDH can be even made specific to certain populations is critical for the future of public health, researchers, government agencies, and the general population. To date and speaking to a high effect, SDHs are an evidence-led science that is factored into all research methodology. Based on the listed information, income, social capital, gender, location, and overall SES are social factors that influence the prevalence of diabetes and its self-management. Therefore, future research and policies must consider the social factors influencing disease as their implications are observable.

Curing diabetes is far beyond human exploration; however, as a result of the efforts of scientific discovery and researchers, individuals living with diabetes can have treatment options to live a healthy life despite the chronic disease. The understanding and application of SDHs in healthcare can be a lasting solution that can reduce the prevalence of diabetes. Healthcare practitioners should focus on understanding how different social factors influence this wide-reaching disease and how they can implement screening methods to identify them. From there, epidemiologists and fellow government agencies should focus on implementing evidence-led strategies to reduce the rates of diabetes within populations and implement inclusive interventions for diverse populations. Although a global perspective on diabetes is challenging and complex, upstream interventions to prevent it can save significant time, provide a better quality of life, and overall a cost-effective solution.

REFERENCES

Asaduzzaman, M., Chowdhury, S., Shahed, J. H., Kafi, M. A. H., Uzzaman, Md. N., Flowra, M. T., & Ahmed, M. M. (2018). Prevalence of Type 2 Diabetes Mellitus Among Urban Bihari Communities in Dhaka, Bangladesh: A Cross-sectional Study in a Minor Ethnic Group. *Cureus.* https://doi.org/10.7759/cureus.2116

Azevedo, M. R., Araújo, C. L. P., Reichert, F. F., Siqueira, F. V., da Silva, M. C., & Hallal, P. C. (2007). Gender differences in leisure-time physical activity. *International Journal of Public Health, 52*(1), 8–15. https://doi.org/10.1007/s00038-006-5062-1

Bärebring, L., Palmqvist, M., Winkvist, A., & Augustin, H. (2020). Gender differences in perceived food healthiness and food avoidance in a Swedish population-based survey: a cross sectional study. *Nutrition Journal, 19*(1). https://doi.org/10.1186/s12937-020-00659-0

Bates, L. M., Hankivsky, O., & Springer, K. W. (2009). Gender and health inequities: A comment on the Final Report of the WHO Commission on the Social Determinants of Health. *Social Science & Medicine, 69*(7), 1002–1004. https://doi.org/10.1016/j.socscimed.2009.07.021

Bernazzani, S. (2016, May). *The Importance of Considering the Social Determinants of Health.* AJMC;https://www.ajmc.com/view/the-importance-of-considering-the-social-determinants-of-health

Bird, Y., Lemstra, M., Rogers, M., & Moraros, J. (2015). The relationship between socioeconomic status/income and prevalence of diabetes and associated conditions: A cross-sectional population-based study in Saskatchewan, Canada. *International Journal for Equity in Health, 14*(1). https://doi.org/10.1186/s12939-015-0237-0

CDC. (2022, April 5). Diabetes Risk Factors. *Centers for Disease Control and Prevention*. https://www.cdc.gov/diabetes/basics/risk-factors.html

Chin, M. H., Cook, S., Jin, L., Drum, M. L., Harrison, J. F., Koppert, J., Thiel, F., Harrand, A. G., Schaefer, C. T., Takashima, H. T., & Chiu, S.-C. . (2001). Barriers to Providing Diabetes Care in Community Health Centers. *Diabetes Care, 24(*2), 268–274. https://doi.org/10.2337/diacare.24.2.268

Diabetes in Africa. (2022). IDF. https://www.idf.org/our-network/regions-members/africa/diabetes-in-africa.html.

Dinca-Panaitescu, S., Dinca-Panaitescu, M., Bryant, T., Daiski, I., Pilkington, B., & Raphael, D. (2011). Diabetes prevalence and income: Results of the Canadian Community Health Survey. *Health Policy, 99*(2), 116–123. https://doi.org/10.1016/j.healthpol.2010.07.018

Ethnicity and type 2 diabetes. (2022). *DiabetesCanadaWebsite.* https://www.diabetes.ca/resources/tools---resources/ethnicity-and-type-2-diabetes

Factors contributing to higher incidence of diabetes for black Americans. (2018, January 8). *National Institutes of Health (NIH).* https://www.nih.gov/news-events/nih-research-matters/factors-contributing-higher-incidence-diabetes-black-americans#:~:text=In%20the%20U.S.%2C%20black%20adults,Mercedes%20R.

Gannon, B., & Roberts, J. (2018). Social capital: exploring the theory and empirical divide. *Empirical Economics, 58*(3), 899–919. https://doi.org/10.1007/s00181-018-1556-y

Gupta, N., Crouse, D. L., & Balram, A. (2020). Individual and community-level income and the risk of diabetes rehospitalization among women and men: a Canadian population-based cohort study. *BMC Public Health, 20*(1). https://doi.org/10.1186/s12889-020-8159-1

Islam, M. M. (2019). Social Determinants of Health and Related Inequalities: Confusion and Implications. *Frontiers in Public Health, 7.* https://doi.org/10.3389/fpubh.2019.00011

Jena, B., Kalra, S., & Yeravdekar, R. (2018). Emotional and psychological needs of people with diabetes. *Indian Journal of Endocrinology and Metabolism, 22*(5), 696. https://doi.org/10.4103/ijem.ijem_579_17

Kooner, J. S., Saleheen, D., Sim, X., Sehmi, J., Zhang, W., Frossard, P., Been, L. F., Chia, K.-S., Dimas, A. S., Hassanali, N., Jafar, T., Jowett, J. B. M., Li, X., Radha, V., Rees, S. D., Takeuchi, F., Young, R., Aung, T., Basit, A., & Chidambaram, M. (2011). Genome-wide association study in individuals of South Asian ancestry identifies six new type 2 diabetes susceptibility loci. *Nature Genetics, 43*(10), 984–989. https://doi.org/10.1038/ng.921

Moradi, Y., Nasehi, M., Asadi-Lari, M., Khamseh, M. E., & Baradaran, H. R. (2017). The relationship between social capital components and control of type 2 diabetes: A path analysis model. *Medical Journal of the Islamic Republic of Iran, 31*(1), 119–123. https://doi.org/10.18869/mjiri.31.21

Muilwijk, M., Nicolaou, M., Qureshi, S. A., Celis-Morales, C., Gill, J. M. R., Sheikh, A., Sattar, N., Beune, E., Jenum, A. K., Stronks, K., & van Valkengoed, I. G. M. (2018). Dietary and physical activity recommendations to prevent type 2 diabetes in South Asian adults: A systematic review. *PLOS ONE, 13*(7), e0200681. https://doi.org/10.1371/journal.pone.0200681

Narayan, K. M. V., & Kanaya, A. M. (2020). Why are South Asians prone to type 2 diabetes? A hypothesis based on underexplored pathways. *Diabetologia, 63*(6), 1103–1109. https://doi.org/10.1007/s00125-020-05132-5

National Center for Biotechnology Information. (2022). Nih.gov. https://www.ncbi.nlm.nih.gov/ *New Research Uncovers Concerning Increases in Youth Living with Diabetes in the U.S.* (2016, January 1). CDC. https://www.cdc.gov/media/releases/2021/p0824-youth-diabetes.html

Pandit, K., Goswami, S., Ghosh, S., Mukhopadhyay, P., & Chowdhury, S. (2012). Metabolic syndrome in South Asians. *Indian Journal of Endocrinology and Metabolism, 16*(1), 44. https://doi.org/10.4103/2230-8210.91187

Peek, M. E., Wagner, J., Tang, H., Baker, D. C., & Chin, M. H. (2011). Self-reported Racial Discrimination in Health Care and Diabetes Outcomes. *Medical Care, 49*(7), 618–625. https://doi.org/10.1097/mlr.0b013e318215d925

Rivera, L. A., Lebenbaum, M., & Rosella, L. C. (2015). The influence of socioeconomic status on future risk for developing Type 2 diabetes in the Canadian population between 2011 and 2022: differential associations by sex. *International Journal for Equity in Health, 14*(1). https://doi.org/10.1186/s12939-015-0245-0

Saeedi, P., Petersohn, I., Salpea, P., Malanda, B., Karuranga, S., Unwin, N., Colagiuri, S., Guariguata, L., Motala, A. A., Ogurtsova, K., Shaw, J. E., Bright, D., & Williams, R. (2019). Global and regional diabetes prevalence estimates for 2019 and projections for 2030 and 2045: Results from the International Diabetes Federation Diabetes Atlas, 9th edition. *Diabetes Research and Clinical Practice, 157*, 107843. https://doi.org/10.1016/j.diabres.2019.107843

Social Determinants of Health. (2016). Cmha.ca. https://ontario.cmha.ca/provincial-policy/social-determinants/#:~:text=In%20Canada%2C%20the%20social%20determinants%20of%20health%20include%3A,Employment%20and%20working%20conditions.%20Food%20insecurity.%20Health%20services

Spanakis, E. K., & Golden, S. H. (2013). Race/Ethnic Difference in Diabetes and Diabetic Complications. *Current Diabetes Reports, 13*(6), 814–823. https://doi.org/10.1007/s11892-013-0421-9

Tang, M., Chen, Y., & Krewski, D. (2003). Gender-related differences in the association between socioeconomic status and self-reported diabetes. *International Journal of Epidemiology, 32*(3), 381–385. https://doi.org/10.1093/ije/dyg075

Temneanu, O. R., Trandafir, L. M., & Purcarea, M. R. (2016). Type 2 diabetes mellitus in children and adolescents: a relatively new clinical problem within pediatric practice. *Journal of Medicine and Life, 9*(3), 235–239. https://www.ncbi.nlm.nih.gov/pmc/articles/PMC5154306/

Westman, E. C. (2021). Type 2 Diabetes Mellitus: A Pathophysiologic Perspective. *Frontiers in Nutrition, 8.* https://doi.org/10.3389/fnut.2021.707371

Winkleby, M. A., Jatulis, D. E., Frank, E., & Fortmann, S. P. (1992). Socioeconomic status and health: how education, income, and occupation contribute to risk factors for cardiovascular disease. *American Journal of Public Health, 82*(6), 816–820. https://doi.org/10.2105/ajph.82.6.816

Worthy, L. D., Lavigne, T., & Romero, F. (2020, July 27). *Socioeconomic Status (SES).* Maricopa.edu; MMOER.https://open.maricopa.edu/ culturepsychology/chapter/socioeconomic-status-ses/

Wu, Y., Ding, Y., Tanaka, Y., & Zhang, W. (2014). Risk Factors Contributing to Type 2 Diabetes and Recent Advances in the Treatment and Prevention. *International Journal of Medical Sciences, 11*(11), 1185–1200. https://doi.org/10.7150/ijms.10001

Yamada, Y., Suematsu, M., Takahashi, N., Okazaki, K., Yasui, H., Hida, T., Uemura, K., Murotani, K., & Kuzuya, M. (2018). Identifying the social capital influencing diabetes control in Japan. *Nagoya Journal of Medical Science, 80*(1), 99–107. https://doi.org/10.18999/nagjms.80.1.99

Zhang, J., Xu, L., Li, J., Sun, L., Qin, W., Ding, G., Wang, Q., Zhu, J., Yu, Z., Xie, S., & Zhou, C. (2019). Gender differences in the association between body mass index and health-related quality of life among adults:a cross-sectional study in Shandong, China. *BMC Public Health, 19*(1). https://doi.org/10.1186/s12889-019-7351-7

CHAPTER 5: VASCULAR COMPLICATIONS OF DIABETES MELLITUS
by Varun Srikanth*, HBHSc

Introduction

Diabetes mellitus (DM) is a disease characterized by a chronic state of hyperglycemia (Luna et al., 2021). There are two primary forms of DM: Type 1 diabetes mellitus (T1DM) and Type 2 diabetes mellitus (T2DM) . In addition, depending on the origin, category, and stage of metabolic dysregulation, a range of physiological complications affecting various organ systems may arise . This chapter will highlight two classes of DM complications: microvascular and macrovascular.

Microvascular complications involve the small blood vessels of the body, like capillaries (Ighodaro & Adeosun, 2017). In diabetic patients, these typically include retinopathy, nephropathy, and neuropathy. In contrast, macrovascular complications involve diseases of the larger blood vessels such as coronary arteries, peripheral arteries, and cerebral arteries. Depending on the stage of the macrovascular complication, associated diseases may range from atherosclerosis to more serious physiological events like myocardial infarction or stroke.

Microvascular Complications

Diabetic Retinopathy

The National Eye Institute (2022) defines diabetic retinopathy as "an eye condition that can cause vision loss and blindness in people [with] diabetes". Diabetic retinopathy primarily affects two regions of the eye: the retina and the macula, and in some cases, both (National Eye Institute, 2022). The retina is a tissue layer in the back of the eye that converts light into neural signals (Addo et al., 2016). The macula is the central region found on the retina that is involved in detailed visual processing (Addo et al., 2016).

There are two main types of diabetic retinopathy: non-proliferative (NPDR) and proliferative (PDR) (Fowler, 2008). Hyperglycemia generally damages the eyes' microvessels, known as retinal capillaries (Fowler, 2008). Weakened capillary walls produce small outpouchings called microaneurysms – indicating the first signs of NPDR (Fowler, 2008). Clinically, these outpouchings present as small scattered dots in the peripheral retina with yellow lipid deposits or hardened fluid known as exudates that emerge due to vessel leakage (Fowler, 2008; American Academy of Ophthalmology, 2018). In addition, ruptured retinal capillaries will cause an outpouring of blood, called a hemorrhage, deep within the retina (Fowler, 2008). Typically, these hemorrhages will present as red dots, often referred to as "dot" or "dot-and-blot" hemorrhages (Fowler, 2008). The natural progression of NPDR is the obstruction of the affected microvessels, which will inevitably damage the nerve fibre (Fowler, 2008). One consequence of a retinal hemorrhage is a build-up of fluid near the macula, known as macular edema, which can severely impede its functioning (Romero-Aroca, 2011). If macular edema is left untreated promptly, permanent blindness may occur (Romero-Aroca, 2011).

PDR unfolds through the continued obstruction, or ischemia, of the microvasculature (Osaadon et al., 2014). Ischemia triggers the retinal cells to release a signalling protein called vascular endothelial growth factor (VEGF), which promotes vascular growth in the retina to circumvent the obstructed vessels. While this may seem physiologically productive, these newly developed vessels are fragile and improperly directed – sometimes even accosting the retina and into the vitreous lining. There are two reasons why this can be problematic: firstly, when we age, the vitreous lining structurally detracts, which strains the newly emerged vessels and causes them to break; and secondly, these new vessels may produce scarring between the vitreous lining and the retina, risking retinal detachment, and by extension, vision loss or blindness.

Diabetic retinopathy is currently the most common microvascular complication of DM (Teo et al., 2021). It is also the fifth leading cause of vision loss and blindness in people with diabetes over fifty (Teo et al., 2021). Moreover, the global prevalence of diabetic retinopathy has been steadily rising; in fact, the International Diabetes Federation predicts the global prevalence of diabetic retinopathy to be over 700 million by 2045 (Fowler, 2008). These statistics require serious consideration because we have an aging global population. While diagnostic and therapeutic tools help identify and reduce DR progression, no cure exists today (Zhang et al., 2018). Therefore, education and awareness are paramount in preventing and reducing DM progression and its associated comorbidities.

Diabetic Nephropathy

The primary role of the kidneys is to remove waste products and excess fluid within the body through millions of filtering units called nephrons (Rayner et al., 2016). Each nephron comprises two structural units: the glomerulus and the tubule (Rayner et al., 2016). The glomerulus is involved in filtering the blood, and the tubule is responsible for releasing needed substances back into the bloodstream while simultaneously removing waste products (DeFronzo et al., 2012). However, diabetic patients may develop diabetic nephropathy (DN), otherwise known as diabetic kidney disease, which impedes the kidneys' ability to filter and remove these waste products (Lim, 2014). As the disease progresses, it will gradually damage the waste filtering system, and when improperly managed, DN may lead to kidney failure (Lim, 2014). Management of

DN in its early stages may involve careful glycemic control and lifestyle changes, but once the patient reaches kidney failure, these efforts become trivial. At this point, the primary treatment options become hemodialysis or renal transplantation (Lim, 2014).

The initial indicator of DN is microalbuminuria: elevated albumin levels in the urine, specifically between 30 mg/day and 299 mg/day (Fowler, 2008; Jong and Curhan, 2006). Albumin is a protein in the blood that plays many vital roles: it aids in muscle development, tissue repair, and fighting infection (Doweiko & Nompleggi, 1991). It also helps manage vascular fluid retention via the maintenance of oncotic pressure (Braswell & Mensack, 2013). In addition, healthy kidneys will aim to excrete waste products; however, diagnostically significant albumin levels in the urine may indicate kidney dysfunction (Comper et al., 2008). If disregarded, microalbuminuria will inevitably progress to albuminuria, where albumin levels exceed 300 mg/day (Fowler, 2008; Jong and Curhan, 2006). Clinicians will typically perform three urine collections because it is estimated that albumin excretion may vary by up to forty percent in diabetics; hence, it is standard for clinicians to collect more than one urine sample to confirm an albuminuria diagnosis (Jong and Curhan, 2006).

DN also triggers several pathological changes in the kidneys. There are several proposed mechanisms, albeit none firmly established. A typical clinical observation is an increased glomerular basement thickness, accompanied by microaneurysm formation (Cade, 2008). The mechanisms leading to the above effects may overlap with those involving diabetic retinopathy, but this requires more investigation.

The seriousness of the condition is compounded by its prevalence in the diabetic patient population. Approximately 20% to 40% of DM patients develop diabetic kidney disease, and both T1DM and T2DM patients can develop this condition, with T2DM patients less likely to progress to end-stage kidney failure (Gheith et al., 2015). Moreover, since there is a greater prevalence of T2DM than T1DM, the former patient population accounts for more than 50% of diabetic patients undergoing hemodialysis. The most effective ways to prevent or slow DN progression is early diagnosis and treatment, consistent lifestyle management, and careful monitoring.

Diabetic Neuropathy

The American Diabetes Association (2007) defines diabetic neuropathy (DNP) as "the presence of symptoms and/or signs of peripheral nerve dysfunction in people with diabetes after the exclusion of other causes." It is a heterogeneous condition involving the pathology of various types of nerves around the body due to chronic exposure to hyperglycemia and high triglyceride levels in the blood (Fowler, 2008). Generally speaking, symptoms can be mild pain and numbness to more intense and persistent pain involving internal organ functionality (National Institute of Diabetes and Digestive and Kidney Diseases (NIDDK), n.d.-a). Similar to diabetic retinopathy and nephropathy, the risk and severity of developing DNP depend on the duration and severity of hyperglycemia, and are contingent on the individuals' genetic profile (Fowler, 2008). Despite these intricacies, certain complications are ubiquitous among diabetic patients. For instance, approximately 50% of DM patients will develop a foot ulcer at some point (Fowler, 2008). Several DNP outcomes also negatively impact one's quality of life, like the increased likelihood of falling and even mental health diagnoses like depression (Hicks & Selvin, 2019).

There are four main types of DNP: peripheral, autonomic, focal, and proximal (Juster-Switlyk & Smith, 2016). Peripheral neuropathy (PNP) is the most common complication of DNP, affecting between one-third to half of all diabetic patients (Juster-Switlyk & Smith, 2016). PNP presents a range of sensory-related symptoms, including loss of pain sensation, tingling, burning, and hyperalgesia (i.e., hypersensitivity and response to pain) (Juster-Switlyk & Smith, 2016). Sensory-related symptoms usually begin at the toes and gradually affect the legs and upper limbs (Juster-Switlyk & Smith, 2016). Clinical examination of PNP typically involves inspection of the feet and a reflex and sensory assessment of physical stimuli like vibration and pinpricks (Tesfaye & Selvarajah, 2012).

Autonomic neuropathy (ANP) is nerve damage of neurons associated with internal organ functionality (Vinik et al., 2003). While ANP is a common complication of DNP and may coexist with PNP, it may also present by itself. Common clinical presentations include resting tachycardia, diminished neurovascular function, and gastroparesis (i.e., delayed gastric emptying). Some symptoms may be physiologically contradictory, but since many organs receive innervation from both the sympathetic and parasympathetic division of the autonomic nervous system, ANP can present as a system-wide disorder.

The third type is focal neuropathies (FNP), which is a condition involving damage to single nerves, most commonly in the upper and lower limbs, head, or torso (NIDDK, n.d.-b). The most common FNPs are entrapment neuropathies, which refer to nerve damage due to compression or irritation (NIDDK, n.d.-b ; Schmid et al., 2020). A well-known example of entrapment neuropathy in diabetic patients is carpal tunnel syndrome, which is a condition that causes numbness or pain in the hand and forearm region due to the compression of the median nerve that travels through the wrist (Werner & Andary, 2011). Several reasons for the high prevalence of carpal tunnel syndrome have been proposed: metabolic dysregulation, edema in the carpal tunnel space, and even diabetic cheiroarthropathy (Vinik et al., 2004).

The fourth type is proximal neuropathy (PNP): a rare form of nerve damage localized to the hip, buttock, or thigh regions and affects only one side of the body (NIDDK, n.d.-c). Like the other neuropathies, the pathophysiology of PNP is not fully understood, but patients have demonstrated gradual improvement over several months or years, though never fully recovering. Diagnostic tools like nerve conduction studies and electromyography (EMG) are typically used. The former checks the rate of electrical signal firing, and the latter shows how responsive the muscles are to the nerves.

Macrovascular Complications

Atherosclerosis

Atherosclerosis is the narrowing of the arterial walls throughout the body and is the primary pathological mechanism leading to macrovascular complications (Fowler, 2008). While the precise mechanisms by which diabetes triggers atherosclerosis are undefined, the association between both conditions is significant. In essence, atherosclerotic plaque formation is believed to result from chronic inflammation and injury to the arterial walls (Cade, 2008). In particular, when the endothelial layer of the artery is damaged, low-density lipoproteins (LDLs) release non-soluble biomolecules called oxidized lipids, which begin to accumulate around this lining (Cade, 2008). Consequently, inflammatory molecules, like monocytes, migrate to these areas and differentiate into macrophages (Cade, 2008). Macrophages then ingest the accumulated oxidized lipids, forming foam cells and triggering a series of cascading steps (Cade, 2008).

These steps primarily involve stimulating a rapid increase of macrophages and attraction of T-lymphocytes, which induces smooth muscle growth in the arterial walls and an accumulation of collagen (Poznyak et al., 2020). The end result of this process is the formation of atherosclerotic lesions with thick layers of connective tissue known as fibrous caps. In diabetic patients, poor glycemic control coupled with high serum levels of adhesion proteins that recruit inflammatory molecules further facilitates foam cell formation and the subsequent cascading response.

Atherosclerosis can be fatal for diabetic patients. Unstable atherosclerotic plaques are at risk of rupturing; if this happens, vascular infarction will occur (Poznyak et al., 2020). In addition, the accumulation of these plaques can result in luminal narrowing, causing metabolic changes and ischemia. When left untreated, there is an increased likelihood of fatal physiological events like myocardial infarction and stroke.

Cardiovascular Disease

Cardiovascular disease (CVD) is a group of disorders of the heart and the vasculature in the body (Nabel, 2003). It is not only the leading cause of death in DM patients but also the highest contributor of healthcare dollars to this patient population, augmenting the burden of this disease (Fowler, 2008). DM patients are at an increased risk of developing CVD as well; in fact, they have a four-fold greater risk of experiencing a non-trivial CVD event when compared to non-diabetics after accounting for risk factors of CVD like age and hypertension (Cade, 2008). Notwithstanding the existence of other risk factors, emerging literature demonstrates that a DM diagnosis is an independent risk factor for CVD (Cade, 2008). Physiological complications like oxidative stress, autonomic neuropathy, and endothelial dysfunction, commonly observed in diabetics, have also been linked to CVD (Leon & Maddox, 2015). While the exact etiological mechanisms are unclear, insulin resistance, hyperglycemia, and atherosclerosis are significant determinants (Huang et al., 2017). Common DM-related CVDs include coronary artery disease, cerebrovascular disease, and peripheral artery disease (Nabel, 2003).

Coronary artery disease (CAD), or ischemic heart disease, is a result of plaque accumulation within the arteries that supply blood to the heart

(CDC, 2021). The gradual accumulation of plaque deposits causes the narrowing of the coronary arteries via atherosclerosis (CDC, 2021). A common symptom of CAD is angina, or chest pain, due to partial or complete obstruction of the coronary arteries; however, an essential indicator of this disease is usually myocardial infarction (MI) (CDC, 2021). Compared to non-diabetic patients who have had an MI in the past, DM patients have a five-time greater risk of a first MI and a two-time greater risk of a recurrent event (Cade, 2008). Furthermore, they have higher mortality following MI and poorer long-term prognoses with CAD (Aronson & Edelman, 2014).

On the other hand, cerebrovascular disease (CBD) involves the pathology of the vessels supplying blood to the brain (Phipps et al., 2012). In experimental stroke models, DM has been shown to increase "cerebral edema, neovascularization, and protease expression", which can compromise the structural integrity of the cerebral vessel walls (Phipps et al., 2012). Moreover, DM increases the likelihood of intra- and extra-cranial atherosclerosis, which may lead to three cerebrovascular events: ischemic stroke, transient ischemic attack, or a hemorrhagic stroke (Balakumar et al., 2016; Cade, 2008). Ischemic stroke results from a thrombus, or blood clot, obstructing blood flow to the brain (Balakumar et al., 2016). A transient ischemic attack also causes an obstruction of blood, but unlike an ischemic stroke, it is only a temporary blockage and does not result in permanent damage (Balakumar et al., 2016). Finally, a hemorrhagic stroke is the rupturing of cerebrovasculature, causing blood to bleed into the brain (Balakumar et al., 2016).

Peripheral artery disease (PAD) is an atherosclerotic occlusive condition that affects the lower extremities (Thiruvoipati et al., 2015). PAD symptoms typically manifest as claudication, cramping, numbness, or pain, but DM patients with PAD are also at an increased risk of MIs and stroke. PAD can be debilitating and cause significant long-term disability.

When hyperglycemia in DM patients is poorly managed, there is a risk of adverse health outcomes. These outcomes may require invasive procedures like endovascular intervention or permanent procedures like an amputation.

Conclusion

This chapter presents a summary of the microvascular and macrovascular complications of DM. When poorly managed, DM can cause severe metabolic changes, life-threatening physiological events, and even death. The burden of DM is significant and requires meticulous effort from clinicians and their patients to reduce the progression of the disease and its associated comorbidities. Awareness and education are critical in taking productive steps forward in prevention and treatment.

REFERENCES

Addo, E., Bamiro, O. A., & Siwale, R. (2016). Anatomy of the Eye and Common Diseases Affecting the Eye. In R. T. Addo (Ed.), *Ocular Drug Delivery: Advances, Challenges and Applications* (pp. 11–25). Springer International Publishing. https://doi.org/10.1007/978-3-319-47691-9_2

American Diabetes Association: Standards of medical care in diabetes—2007 [Position Statement]. Diabetes Care 30:S4-S41, 2007

Aronson, D., & Edelman, E. R. (2014). Coronary Artery Disease and Diabetes Mellitus. *Cardiology Clinics, 32*(3), 439–455. https://doi.org/10.1016/j.ccl.2014.04.001

Balakumar, P., Maung-U, K., & Jagadeesh, G. (2016). Prevalence and prevention of cardiovascular disease and diabetes mellitus. *Pharmacological Research, 113,* 600–609. https://doi.org/10.1016/j.phrs.2016.09.040

Braswell, C., & Mensack, S. (2013). Chapter 11—Supportive Care of the Poisoned Patient. In M. E. Peterson & P. A. Talcott (Eds.), *Small Animal Toxicology (Third Edition)* (pp. 85–124). W.B. Saunders. https://doi.org/10.1016/B978-1-4557-0717-1.00011-9

Cade, W. T. (2008). Diabetes-Related Microvascular and Macrovascular Diseases in the Physical Therapy Setting. *Physical Therapy, 88*(11), 1322–1335. https://doi.org/10.2522/ptj.20080008

CDC. (2021, July 19). *Coronary Artery Disease | cdc.gov.* Centers for Disease Control and Prevention. https://www.cdc.gov/heartdisease/coronary_ad.html

Comper, W. D., Hilliard, L. M., Nikolic-Paterson, D. J., & Russo, L. M. (2008). Disease-dependent mechanisms of albuminuria. *American Journal of Physiology-Renal Physiology, 295*(6), F1589–F1600. https://doi.org/10.1152/ajprenal.00142.2008

DeFronzo, R. A., Davidson, J. A., & Del Prato, S. (2012). The role of the kidneys in glucose homeostasis: A new path towards normalizing glycaemia. *Diabetes, Obesity and Metabolism, 14*(1), 5–14. https://doi.org/10.1111/j.1463-1326.2011.01511.x

National Institute of Diabetes and Digestive and Kidney Diseases. (n.d.-a). *Diabetic Neuropathy Diabetic Neuropathy.* Retrieved July 8, 2022, from https://www.niddk.nih.gov/health-information/diabetes/overview/preventing-problems/nerve-damage-diabetic-neuropathies

National Institute of Diabetes and Digestive and Kidney Diseases. (n.d.-b). *Focal Neuropathies | NIDDK.* Retrieved July 8, 2022, from https://www.niddk.nih.gov/health-information/diabetes/overview/preventing-problems/nerve-damage-diabetic-neuropathies/focal-neuropathies

National Institute of Diabetes and Digestive and Kidney Diseases. (n.d.-c). *Proximal Neuropathy | NIDDK.* Retrieved July 8, 2022, from https://www.niddk.nih.gov/health-information/diabetes/overview/preventing-problems/nerve-damage-diabetic-neuropathies/proximal-neuropathy

National Eye Institute. (2022). *Diabetic Retinopathy.* Retrieved July 8, 2022, from https://www.nei.nih.gov/learn-about-eye-health/eye-conditions-and-diseases/diabetic-retinopathy

Doweiko, J. P., & Nompleggi, D. J. (1991). Reviews: Role of Albumin in Human Physiology and Pathophysiology. *Journal of Parenteral and Enteral Nutrition, 15*(2), 207–211. https://doi.org/10.1177/0148607191015002207

Fowler, M. J. (2008). Microvascular and Macrovascular Complications of Diabetes. *Clinical Diabetes, 26*(2), 77–82. https://doi.org/10.2337/diaclin.26.2.77

Gheith, O., Farouk, N., Nampoory, N., Halim, M. A., & Al-Otaibi, T. (2015). Diabetic kidney disease: World wide difference of prevalence and risk factors. *Journal of Nephropharmacology, 5*(1), 49–56.

Hicks, C. W., & Selvin, E. (2019). Epidemiology of Peripheral Neuropathy and Lower Extremity Disease in Diabetes. *Current Diabetes Reports, 19*(10), 86. https://doi.org/10.1007/s11892-019-1212-8

Huang, D., Refaat, M., Mohammedi, K., Jayyousi, A., Al Suwaidi, J., & Abi Khalil, C. (2017). Macrovascular Complications in Patients with Diabetes and Prediabetes. *BioMed Research International, 2017*, e7839101. https://doi.org/10.1155/2017/7839101

Ighodaro, O., & Adeosun, A. (2017). Vascular Complication in Diabetes Mellitus. *The Lancet Diabetes & Endocrinology, i*, 1–3. https://doi.org/10.31031/GJEM.2017.01.000506

Jong, P. E. de, & Curhan, G. C. (2006). Screening, Monitoring, and Treatment of Albuminuria: Public Health Perspectives. *Journal of the American Society of Nephrology, 17*(8), 2120–2126. https://doi.org/10.1681/ASN.2006010097

Juster-Switlyk, K., & Smith, A. G. (2016). Updates in diabetic peripheral neuropathy. *F1000Research, 5*, F1000 Faculty Rev-738. https://doi.org/10.12688/f1000research.7898.1

Leon, B. M., & Maddox, T. M. (2015). Diabetes and cardiovascular disease: Epidemiology, biological mechanisms, treatment recommendations and future research. *World Journal of Diabetes, 6*(13), 1246–1258. https://doi.org/10.4239/wjd.v6.i13.1246

Lim, A. K. (2014). Diabetic nephropathy – complications and treatment. *International Journal of Nephrology and Renovascular Disease, 7,* 361–381. https://doi.org/10.2147/IJNRD.S40172

Luna, R., Talanki Manjunatha, R., Bollu, B., Jhaveri, S., Avanthika, C., Reddy, N., Saha, T., & Gandhi, F. (2021). A Comprehensive Review of Neuronal Changes in Diabetics. *Cureus.* https://doi.org/10.7759/cureus.19142

American Academy of Ophthalmology. (2018, January 8). *Microaneurysms.* https://www.aao.org/image/microaneurysms-4

Nabel, E. G. (2003). Cardiovascular Disease. *New England Journal of Medicine, 349*(1), 60–72. https://doi.org/10.1056/NEJMra035098

Osaadon, P., Fagan, X. J., Lifshitz, T., & Levy, J. (2014). A review of anti-VEGF agents for proliferative diabetic retinopathy. *Eye, 28*(5), 510–520. https://doi.org/10.1038/eye.2014.13

Phipps, M. S., Jastreboff, A. M., Furie, K., & Kernan, W. N. (2012). The Diagnosis and Management of Cerebrovascular Disease in Diabetes. *Current Diabetes Reports, 12*(3), 314–323. https://doi.org/10.1007/s11892-012-0271-x

Poznyak, A., Grechko, A. V., Poggio, P., Myasoedova, V. A., Alfieri, V., & Orekhov, A. N. (2020). The Diabetes Mellitus–Atherosclerosis Connection: The Role of Lipid and Glucose Metabolism and Chronic Inflammation. *International Journal of Molecular Sciences, 21*(5), 1835. https://doi.org/10.3390/ijms21051835

Rayner, H., Thomas, M., & Milford, D. (2016). Kidney Anatomy and Physiology. *Understanding Kidney Diseases, 1–*10. https://doi. org/10.1007/978-3-319-23458-8_1

Romero-Aroca, P. (2011). Managing diabetic macular edema: The leading cause of diabetes blindness. *World Journal of Diabetes, 2*(6), 98–104. https://doi.org/10.4239/wjd.v2.i6.98

Schmid, A. B., Fundaun, J., & Tampin, B. (2020). Entrapment neuropathies: A contemporary approach to pathophysiology, clinical assessment, and management. *PAIN Reports, 5*(4), e829. https://doi. org/10.1097/PR9.0000000000000829

Teo, Z. L., Tham, Y.-C., Yu, M., Chee, M. L., Rim, T. H., Cheung, N., Bikbov, M. M., Wang, Y. X., Tang, Y., Lu, Y., Wong, I. Y., Ting, D. S. W., Tan, G. S. W., Jonas, J. B., Sabanayagam, C., Wong, T. Y., & Cheng, C.-Y. (2021). Global Prevalence of Diabetic Retinopathy and Projection of Burden through 2045. *Ophthalmology, 128*(11), 1580–1591. https://doi. org/10.1016/j.ophtha.2021.04.027

Tesfaye, S., & Selvarajah, D. (2012). Advances in the epidemiology, pathogenesis and management of diabetic peripheral neuropathy. *Diabetes/Metabolism Research and Reviews, 28*(S1), 8–14. https://doi. org/10.1002/dmrr.2239

Thiruvoipati, T., Kielhorn, C. E., & Armstrong, E. J. (2015). Peripheral artery disease in patients with diabetes: Epidemiology, mechanisms, and outcomes. *World Journal of Diabetes, 6*(7), 961–969. https://doi.org/10.4239/wjd.v6.i7.961

Vinik, A. I., Maser, R. E., Mitchell, B. D., & Freeman, R. (2003). Diabetic Autonomic Neuropathy. *Diabetes Care, 26*(5), 1553–1579. https://doi.org/10.2337/diacare.26.5.1553

Vinik, A., Mehrabyan, A., Colen, L., & Boulton, A. (2004). Focal Entrapment Neuropathies in Diabetes. *Diabetes Care, 27*(7), 1783–1788. https://doi.org/10.2337/diacare.27.7.1783

Werner, R. A., & Andary, M. (2011). Electrodiagnostic evaluation of carpal tunnel syndrome. *Muscle & Nerve, 44*(4), 597–607. https://doi.org/10.1002/mus.22208

Zhang, H. W., Zhang, H., Grant, S. J., Wan, X., & Li, G. (2018). Single herbal medicine for diabetic retinopathy. *Cochrane Database of Systematic Reviews, 2018*(12), https://doi.org/10.1002/14651858.CD007939.p

CHAPTER 6: A SYSTEMATIC REVIEW OF TRENDS IN DIABETES - RISKS, CHALLENGES, AND RESEARCH ETHICS IMPACTING HEALTH OUTCOMES FOR INDIGENOUS POPULATIONS IN CANADA

by Lydia C Rehman*, HBSc, MPH(c)

Abstract: Diabetes is a major public health issue with increasing concern. Indigenous peoples in Canada have higher rates of type 2 diabetes than that of non-Indigenous peoples. However, research is lacking on the health literacy and knowledge that health professionals hold about barriers and disparities within the Canadian healthcare system. Health care professionals hold the power to evaluate/communicate medical information to patients to reduce the diabetes disease burden, and understanding health literacy is significant to reducing systemic inequities for Indigenous peoples. Poor health status and incidence/prevalence of diabetes in Indigenous populations is result from colonialism, the weaponization of health, historical trauma and racism, structural barriers, and the lack of Indigenous-led research. This paper aims to understand the increasing burdens, disparities, and morbidities surrounding Indigenous peoples and diabetes.

Key Words: Indigenous Health, Diabetes, Historical Trauma & Colonialism, Culturally Safe Care, Decolonized Research Methodologies

Methods: This research is conducted via systematic literature review, while utilizing peer-reviewed resources derived within PubMed, International Journal for Indigenous Health, SCOPUS, Web of Science and other primary peer-reviewed sources of relevance. The keywords used in the database search strategy include: *Indigenous* OR *First Nation* OR *Canada* OR *Diabetes* OR *Health Outcomes* OR *Management* OR *Community-Based Participation* OR *Colonialism* OR *Cultural Safety*

Ethical Considerations/Limiting Factors: When the term "Indigenous peoples" is used, it should be denoted that the term is not homogenous. It recognizes that Indigenous peoples consist of First Nations, Metis, and Inuit people's status/non-status and off-reserve, with distinct/unique languages, cultures, communities, histories & traditions. This systematic literature review will be written in an ethical manner, with reflection on Indigenous realities and respect for cultural integrity by maintaining cultural authenticity, acknowledging sources of Indigenous information, using culturally appropriate language and exerting caution when discussing trauma. It is acknowledged that the ample literature that exists is not within the First Nations OCAP principles, Metis, and Inuit data sovereignty/ethics protocols in an articulate manner, which is highlighted in the context of diabetes research.

Discussions: This paper will further discuss the burden of diabetes, management of diabetes, and challenges for Indigenous populations. Likewise, it will discuss the barriers within research itself-surrounding the ethics of Indigenous health research .

Conclusions: Disparities within Canada need to continue to be addressed with the increased presence of Indigenous traditional knowledge and healing practices. Western medicine is not the only type of medicine that exists and supports the integration of Indigenous healing, and knowledge in an integrated healthcare system only serves to advance Indigenous health, reduce disease burdens associated with diabetes, and to further strengthen Indigenous people's right to self-determination and sovereignty. One question that has derived from the synthesis of the literature is the question of, how is health research working to improve the lives of First Nations, Metis and Inuit peoples with the burden of diabetes, if research is not in ethical considerations of the respective communities.

Introduction

Poor health status, incidence, and prevalence of Type 2 diabetes mellitus (T2DM) in First Nations, Metis, and Inuit populations is the direct result of colonialism, the weaponization of health, historical trauma, racism, structural barriers, and the lack of Indigenous-led research. It is suggested that the residential school system is directly correlated to the increasing incidence of diabetes, as exposure to restricted calories creates metabolic changes within the body, leading to an increased risk for obesity and chronic disease such as diabetes (Mosby & Galloway, 2017). One projection suggests that between 2000-2030 there will be a 214% increase in T2DM in Indigenous populations (Cordier et al., 2020). As of 2022, T2DM affects Indigenous populations at 3-5 times the rate compared to non-Indigenous populations in Canada (Wicklow et al., 2021; IHE, 2017). Within First Nations communities, T2DM is higher in females than males, whereas the rate of T2DM in non-Indigenous communities is highest in men (Cordier et al., 2020). Indigenous populations have higher rates of diabetes complications including "neuropathy, retinopathy, nephropathy, macrovascular disease, and limb amputation" (IHE,2017). Many of these complications result from being diagnosed late or Indigenous patients having decreased access to treatment options. Additionally, First Nations and other groups of Indigenous populations are less likely to achieve standardized care, including the testing and measurement of glycated hemoglobin (HbA1c) and retinal screening (IHE, 2017). The overarching result is that First Nations have higher hospitalization rates and visits to the emergency department for diabetes-related complications (IHE, 2017).

Due to colonialism, and the historical relationships influenced by the Canadian government, Indigenous peoples are more likely to have complexities in managing diabetes, as accessing care is not without its challenges and barriers. Indigenous populations with T2DM face marginalization, discrimination, and racism within healthcare policy, and throughout the healthcare system. One of the many challenges of diabetes management resulting in complications includes a lack of access to private insurance for diabetes medication (IHE, 2017). Similarly, in one study, many of the Indigenous participants with T2DM felt as if they were being experimented on through the push of medication. Coping with long lineups and wait times can be difficult. Many individuals are exhausted by the power imbalances between healthcare providers and patients. Providers do not take the time to develop meaningful relationships with their patients; doctors also frequently assume that patients understand how to manage diabetes through medication. Further, there are physician shortages and accessioning care within smaller/rural communities is not without its difficulties. Indigenous patients fear using Western healthcare systems, as much of the current system is culturally unsafe (Jacklin et al., 2017).

Risk Factors, Interventions and an Overview of T2DM, Indigenous Children, Pregnant Women, Environmental Contaminants

According to one study, researchers found that the rates of T2DM and obesity in Indigenous children in Canada are among the highest globally (Crawford et al., 2019). An increase in T2DM is typically observed with increased rates of obesity, genetic and different social/environmental factors. As previously mentioned, the main drivers of the "obesity epidemic" specific to Indigenous children are settler-colonialism, systemic poverty, and land displacement (Crawford et al., 2019). One of the current barriers affecting prevention is the lack of culturally safe, trauma-informed interventions/health promotion tools that incorporate Indigenous worldviews and traditional knowledge (Crawford et al., 2019). Currently, 50 percent of T2DM in Canada occurs in populations of Indigenous youth. In addition, the onset of diabetes predisposes Indigenous youth to other comorbidities and complexities such as cardiovascular disease (Crawford et al., 2019). Research suggests that First Nations youth diagnosed with diabetes before the age of 20 are at an increased risk of developing renal disease and have a higher likelihood of higher mortality rates than non-First Nations youth.

Current interventions need to be outlined as the rise in obesity and T2DM in youth carries significant health outcomes. Further, without active interventions that are Indigenous-led and meet the specific needs of Indigenous populations, health outcomes of diabetes will likely result in increased complications. A great example to highlight best practices is the Kahnawake Schools Diabetes Prevention Project, developed through a partnership with the Mohawk community of Kahnawake. This project was developed to intervene and prevent the increase in obesity in children (IHE, 2017). The program is community-based and provided to elementary schools through measures of building community through health promotion of physical exercise/activity and healthy eating. This project used a holistic approach, incorporating traditional knowledge and community voices in promoting health and well-being for their community (IHE, 2017). While other Indigenous-led projects exist, there is not enough to meet the diverse needs of Indigenous populations across Canada. Future interventions should use the existing frameworks and programs to develop culturally safe health promotion and prevention initiatives that are Indigenous-led.

As previously stated, a clear health gap exists for Indigenous communities compared to non-Indigenous communities, as colonialism is a driving force behind the health outcomes associated with various chronic diseases such as diabetes (Voaklander et al., 2020). The rate of diabetes in Indigenous women compared to non-Indigenous women is 2-3 times higher (Zuk et al., 2021). According to a study, Status First Nations pregnant women are twice as likely to be hospitalized than non-First Nations women. Indigenous women are at high risk for developing gestational diabetes mellitus (GDM). Typically, within the third trimester of pregnancy for women, it can be observed that there is an evident increase in insulin sensitivity. This insensitivity is a driving cause of GDM, causing women without pre-existing T2DM to develop while pregnant (Zuk et al., 2021). Colonialism is again the largest contributor to the development of T2DM. Unfavourable outcomes of social determinants of health such as income, education, employment, and housing are also barriers to successfully managing T2DM (Voaklander et al., 2020). Much of the current care models are derived from western epistemologies of healthcare and medicine (Voaklander et al., 2020). Interventions to assist in preventing diabetes in pregnant women should be designed and facilitated by Indigenous women, and communities (Voaklander et al., 2020). These programs should ensure Indigenous self-determination in healing and healthcare.

Lastly, there is also evidence that suggests environmental factors are correlated with the onset of T2DM. It is suggested that populations that rely on fish, and marine species within their diets, have higher rates of exposure to metals and persistent organic pollutants (POPs) (Cordier et al., 2020). Researchers compared sample populations between an Inuit and Cree community and previous studies to look at Indigenous populations that frequently consume fish and the level of exposure to metals such as mercury and other organic pollutants. The study found an association between POP exposure and the prevalence of T2DM. Further, within the Nituuchischaayihtitaau Aschii—Multi-Community Environment-Health Study, researchers explored the association between T2DM in First Nations women and environmental exposures to organochlorine pesticides, which include: "dichlorodiphenyltrichloroethane (DDT), and dichlorodiphenyldichloroethylene (DDE)" (Zuk et al., 2021). Overall another association between environmental pollutants and the onset of T2DM was found; however, future research in this area is warranted, as environment and climate change can be analyzed as social determinants of health (Zuk et al., 2021).

The Role of Ethics in Diabetes Research for Indigenous Populations: Reflecting through the OCAP Principles™

This section of the paper, will highlight the First Nations Information Governance Center's OCAP principles and then use them to highlight their role in diabetes research involving Indigenous peoples. Western research methodologies involving Indigenous peoples have reinforced social, physical, psychological, and cultural harms (FNIGC, 2020). First Nations peoples have been subject to much research and have had their data collected and analyzed, which have worked to create harm for communities. Much of the data collected is derived and analyzed from western methodologies and researchers who are not actually interested in the priorities of First Nations communities (FNIGC, 2020). Administrative data tends to be collected without the knowledge of communities and then accessed by the government and researchers within academic institutions (FNIGC, 2020). Many researchers have guilted communities into believing a narrative that "without this research being conducted, your community will not thrive." Many of these harms have included researchers entering a community to benefit their own research without establishing a meaningful relationship (FNIGC, 2020). Much of the data collected has been used to create harmful stereotypes and false narratives about Indigenous communities.

Researchers have also fraudulently misused traditional Indigenous knowledge on medicines and technology to patent for economic, personal, and commercial gains (FNIGC, 2020). Overall Western institutions have worked to harm Indigenous communities through colonial assertions manifested through western research methodologies and epistemologies within qualitative and quantitative research. Likewise, much of the data collected from research studies were never made accessible nor in ownership of the Indigenous communities themselves. However, due to the continued efforts of Indigenous researchers, organizations, and allied scholars, Indigenous self-determination and sovereignty in research are becoming more prominent and ensured. Indigenous self-determination in research and policy ensures that many of the harms caused to the community by Western institutions through research activities, will not continue to be perpetuated. A fantastic example of a data sovereignty strategy plan is the mission of the First Nations Information Governance Center (FNIGC, 2020) and the creation of the Ownership, Possession, Control principles (OCAP™).

These principles highlight the necessary ethics, surrounding research involving First Nations communities. The principles can be understood within the table below:

Ownership	This principle refers to how a community chooses to have a relationship to Indigenous / cultural knowledge, data and information. The community owns the information.
Control	This is the right of First Nations and their communities to be able to control information and data. This can include how data is collected, utilized and overall managed. Communities may also devise plans on how to disclose and destroy data.
Possession	Reflects stewardship over the data that is collected and produced. They protect the ownership and control of the data.
Access	First Nations must be able to have access to the data that is about them. They should also be able to be the decision makers on who can access collected data.

Using all of these principles, and understanding of Indigenous research ethics, applying the execution of these community protocols to current literature is essential in highlighting the barriers that continue to exist within western research methodologies.The OCAP principles can be applied to address the strengths and weaknesses of Indigenous research ethics specific to diabetes research involving Indigenous populations.

 For example, in Jacklin et al. (2017), the authors gather the healthcare experiences of Indigenous peoples living with T2DM In Canada. While this paper highlights many of the challenges of managing diabetes, as well as the Indigenous-specific determinants of health that directly affect health outcomes of diabetes. To carry out this qualitative research, the researchers used purposeful sampling to recruit Indigenous peoples with diabetes to participate in a series of five focus groups. Three of the focus groups were First Nations communities. Something notable within this paper is that they state that "Indigenous ways of knowing and sharing were honoured" but failed to note any consultation with elders, traditional knowledge keepers, and community in the design of this research project. This lack of inclusion of community perspective highlights Western research approaches and how barriers continue to remain consistent. Further, this project is considered "community-based", but the only community-based practice described in the research was ensuring that community members confirm the data interpretation. This paper fails to state the benefit and meaningful relationship built prior to conducting the study, and there is no emphasis on this study being Indigenous-led. This study does not articulate any of the OCAP principles. Lastly, First Nations' experiences of healthcare in the management of diabetes are being collected and thematically analyzed, yet there is no mention of how communities will be able to access this data. Furthermore, they have no control over other organizations that can freely access their data (Jacklin et al., 2017). These are the many factors limiting health research. Given the burden of diabetes and the experiences of Indigenous populations within the healthcare system, research methods need to honour Indigenous worldviews. Indigenous research ethics, specific to the group being researched (First Nations, Metis, Inuit) should fall in line with the community/population protocols for conducting research.

Solutions, Cultural Safety, and Indigenous Self-Determination in the Management of Diabetes

The most productive solution to addressing the healthcare gap for Indigenous populations and the management of diabetes is ensuring access to culturally safe care that respects and honours Indigenous worldviews and knowledge in healthcare is made available. The 2015 Truth and Reconciliation final summary report includes a call to action (22) which clearly states "We call upon those who can affect change within the Canadian health-care system to recognize the value of aboriginal healing practices and use them in the treatment of aboriginal patients in collaboration with Aboriginal healers and elders where requested by Aboriginal patients" (TRC, 2015). This is necessary for healing and promotion with the onset of T2DM. The literature highlights that Indigenous participants in various studies were satisfied when cultural interventions were available. This includes a health education framework where health educators provide information about the management of diabetes to patients. Further, group interventions are also valued, as Indigenous participants can take what is known as a chronic disease of "diabetes" and build a community as a means of wellness and healing. Likewise, having an intervention of shared medical care, where health professionals and traditional healers, elders, and knowledge holders share a meal while providing patients with the "nutritional, psychological and spiritual" support necessary to help them cope with T2DM (Tremblay et al., 2020). To reiterate, the inequities that exist for Indigenous communities compared to non-Indigenous communities are rooted in sociocultural factors. Understanding health from the perspective of Indigenous peoples is more critical to health and well-being than just managing a chronic disease like diabetes (IHE, 2017). Overall, research shows that cultural interventions, Indigneours workforce interventions, and Indigenous self-determination in the Canadian healthcare system are required to make structural changes to create better health outcomes for managing diabetes.

REFERENCES

Cordier, S., Anassour-Laouan-Sidi, E., Lemire, M., Costet, N., Lucas, M., & Ayotte, P. (2020). Association between exposure to persistent organic pollutants and mercury, and glucose metabolism in two Canadian Indigenous populations. *Environmental Research, 184,* 109345–109345. https://doi.org/10.1016/j.envres.2020.109345

Crawford, Sims, E. D., Wang, K.-W., Youssef, M., Nadarajah, A., Rivas, A., Banfield, L., Thabane, L., & Samaan, M. C. (2019). Traditional knowledge-based lifestyle interventions in the prevention of obesity and type 2 diabetes in Indigenous children in Canada: a systematic review protocol. *Systematic Reviews, 8(*1), 69–69. https://doi.org/10.1186/s13643-019-0961-4

First Nations Information Governance Center (FNIGC) 2020 https://achh.ca/wp-content/uploads/2018/07/OCAP_FNIGC.pdfn

Diabetes Care and Management in Indigenous Populations in Canada: A Pan-Canadian Policy Roundtable. (2017). Institute of Health Economics.

Jacklin, Ly, A., Calam, B., Green, M., Walker, L., & Crowshoe, L. (2016). An Innovative Sequential Focus Group Method for Investigating Diabetes Care Experiences With Indigenous Peoples in Canada. *International Journal of Qualitative Methods, 15*(1), 160940691667496–. https://doi.org/10.1177/1609406916674965

Mosby, & Galloway, T. (2017). "Hunger was never absent": How residential school diets shaped current patterns of diabetes among Indigenous peoples in Canada. *Canadian Medical Association Journal (CMAJ), 189*(32), E1043–E1045. https://doi.org/10.1503/cmaj.170448

Tremblay, Graham, J., Porgo, T. V., Dogba, M. J., Paquette, J.-S., Careau, E., & Witteman, H. O. (2020). Improving Cultural Safety of Diabetes Care in Indigenous Populations of Canada, Australia, New Zealand and the United States: A Systematic Rapid Review. *Canadian Journal of Diabetes, 44*(7), 670–678. https://doi.org/10.1016/j.jcjd.2019.11.006

Truth and Reconciliation Commission of Canada, "Truth and Reconciliation Commission of Canada: Calls to Action," *Exhibits,* accessed July 8, 2022, https://exhibits.library.utoronto.ca/items/show/2420.

Voaklander, Rowe, S., Sanni, O., Campbell, S., Eurich, D., & Ospina, M. B. (2020). Prevalence of diabetes in pregnancy among Indigenous women in Australia, Canada, New Zealand, and the USA: a systematic review and meta-analysis. *The Lancet Global Health, 8*(5), e681–e698. https://doi.org/10.1016/S2214-109X(20)30046-2

Wicklow, B., Dart, A., McKee, J., Griffiths, A., Malik, S., Quoquat, S., & Bruce, S. (2021). Experiences of First Nations adolescents living with type 2 diabetes: a focus group study. *Canadian Medical Association Journal (CMAJ), 193*(12), E403–E409. https://doi.org/10.1503/cmaj.201685

Zuk, A., Liberda, E. N., & Tsuji, L. J. S. (2021). Environmental contaminants and the disproportionate prevalence of type-2 diabetes mellitus among Indigenous Cree women in James Bay Quebec, Canada. *Scientific Reports, 11*(1), 24050–24050. https://doi.org/10.1038/s41598-021-03065-6

CHAPTER 7: DIABETES FROM THE PERSPECTIVE OF A HEALTHCARE PROFESSIONAL

by Harshita Saxena*, RN, BScN

Diabetes mellitus (T1DM, T2DM) is a chronic illness impacting many people's lives globally. One in four Canadians is either prediabetic, undiagnosed, or living with diabetes (RNAO, 2020). As a registered nurse and healthcare practitioner, I often interact with patients who have recently been diagnosed with diabetes or have been living with the chronic disease for a while. This chapter will discuss my diabetic patient encounters, the role of nurses in providing care to patients with diabetes, and the barriers to diabetes management – including access to care – and outline the future of diabetes management.

Role of Nurses in the Management of Diabetes

As healthcare professionals, we often work with T1DM and T2DM patients. who are diagnosed with T1DM (autoimmune) or T2DM (later onset and linked with a metabolic disorder like obesity). I have worked as a nurse for almost 1.5 years. I have worked with multiple patients recently diagnosed with diabetes, who developed diabetes during hospitalization or have been living with it for a while. Most of patients with T1DM are very familiar with managing their diabetes, as they have been doing this since childhood. They are well aware of symptoms of hypoglycemia (low blood sugar) and hyperglycemia (high blood sugar) and are acknowledged in carbohydrate counting (counting the number of grams of carbohydrates in a particular meal), and the administration of insulin. In contrast, T2DM patients are unable to look after themselves due to various barriers to optimal healthcare or simply ignore the signs and symptoms presented by their bodies. Nurses are a critical component in assisting patients with the education and management of their diabetes.

Nurses are educators who assist patients in understanding the signs and symptoms of hypo/hyperglycemia, as well as other diabetes-related symptoms. Nurses thoroughly explain the treatment plan initiated by the physician and ensure that patients are aware of the oral medications and insulin injections. Nurses also teach patients about carb counting, how to check blood glucose, and self-inject insulin. Nurses in primary care provide education on primary, secondary and tertiary prevention to prevent or treat/manage diabetes. Primary prevention aims to prevent a disease/condition from happening by relying on education awareness, opting for healthier lifestyles, and up-to-date immunizations. Secondary prevention targets earlier disease detection; for example, by getting tested to make sure one is not suffering from an ailment. Finally, tertiary prevention focuses on rehabilitation activities and how a disease can be prevented from progressing after a patient has been diagnosed (Kisling & Das, 2022).

Occupational health nurses teach patients how to manage a healthy lifestyle with a diabetes diagnosis. There are also diabetes specialist nurses that are primarily trained to provide knowledge and possess skills to take care of patients diagnosed with diabetes. They play an important role in diabetes education. Endocrinologists and endocrinology nurse practitioners are responsible for diagnosing and treating patients who have T1DM & T2DM. For bedside nurses duties include frequent blood sugar checks, calculating insulin needs based on a sliding scale, monitoring carb counting, and ensuring the patient is eating properly. These complications may include necrosis in the limbs, numbness in the lower extremities, and vision changes. Physicians and NPs rely on nurse assessments to provide treatment plans for patients, like determining the dosage of oral medications. For newly diagnosed diabetic patients, nurses assist patients in understanding the importance of healthier lifestyles and stress management. Nurses also play an essential role in helping patients adjust to their new diagnoses. Dealing with diabetes can psychologically impact the patient, and nurses are:

- a great source of emotional support for struggling patients;

- provide a safe space for open communication; and

- are patient advocates.

Many patients complain of diabetes as a burden and an overwhelming process, as they have to frequently check blood sugars throughout the day, which they find challenging to manage. Many children feel inferior to kids who do not have diabetes, as they have to control their cravings and cannot eat as other kids would typically eat. Overall, the psychological implications of going through symptoms of diabetes, dealing with its associated complications, and in extreme cases, undergoing amputation have significant impacts on quality of life.

Barriers within Healthcare for Diabetic Patients

All chronic conditions carry diverse barriers that influence a disease's health outcomes or prevent patients from managing their conditions efficiently. Moreover, effective diabetes management is complicated and hampered by various socio-economic factors, including the individual, community, and health system levels (Pract, 2016). Barriers range from limited access to health care centers, poor health literacy in understanding their diagnosis, unawareness or avoidance of diabetes symptoms, not maintaining regular healthcare checkups, and lack of cultural competency among health care workers (Pract, 2016).

Working with diabetic patients, I have realized there are several factors that contribute to patients being able to manage their diabetes well. Some contributing factors include a lack of knowledge on diabetes, not enough awareness in the community on symptoms, a lack of motivation to make lifestyle changes, stigma around the disease, financial burden, inability to access health care resources, and improper federal funding. Many newly diagnosed patients with diabetes are usually unaware of the signs and symptoms of hypo/hyperglycemia, which prolongs them from seeking timely medical attention. There are also not enough primary preventative measures that promote community engagement to raise awareness about diabetes; this results in an increase in prediabetics. Finally, many patients find it difficult to manage their new diagnosis due to a lack of support from family members or busy work schedules. Thus, patients need to possess self-efficacy skills to better self-manage diabetes.

Next, financial constraints impede patients from eating the recommended diet, and inability to buy the necessary treatment supplies like blood glucose strips (BGS), glucometers, and insulin. Many patients are also not covered through insurance, and various insurance companies will not cover all clinical tests like HbA1c for diabetes supplies leaving these patients with unaffordable bills and treatment. In recent conversations with diabetic patients, some share that the lifelong commitment to diabetes can be overwhelming to manage and deal with. Similarly, patients who travel as part of their profession find it difficult to stick to a prescribed/suggested diet by a healthcare provider. Moreover, many restaurants do not have nutritional information in the menu or share information about carbohydrates, protein and fat ratios in the meals served, further adding to the challenge of self-management.

We also get patients who often neglect the signs and symptoms they experience, thereby delaying treatment. This aggravates the diabetes symptoms, sometimes to a point where the patients have to undergo amputation of limbs. Another barrier to optimal care is understaffing, as nurses might not be able to reach the patients on time. For example, during meal times in hospitals, some patients start eating before the nurse has checked their blood glucose despite knowing it must be confirmed before eating. This leads to inaccurate BG results later and incorrect insulin doses administered at times. In addition, if a patient was having a hypo- or hyperglycemic episode, it might not be caught early as the nurse was busy with other patient duties. It should also be noted that some communities, namely BIPOC communities, do not have equal access to healthcare. Therefore, the government should provide feasible solutions to ensure that all populations with T1DM/T2DM have the necessary resources to prevent and manage diabetes.

Another factor that impacts in-hospital patient care for people with diabetes is overcrowded and loud hallways. There are medical emergencies, multiple staff members working, loud noises of the medical devices like IV poles, PCA pumps, dialysis machines, and multiple patients within one room. All of which increase patient stress levels, which is also co-related to elevated blood sugar levels. Managing diabetes takes much self-control, discipline, patience, and willingness to adapt. Given this disease burden, there are existing mental health services specific to diabetes, and this programming should be expanded and accessible for all diabetic patients to cope. Patients should also be taught about smoking cessation, lowering alcohol intake, and lowering cholesterol levels as it helps patients prevent diabetes, enhances their quality of life, and helps reduce costs to the federal budget (Asif, 2014). With T1DM, it can be challenging to manage physical activity, as patients have to always monitor their blood sugar levels. However, this can be managed with proper education on how much carbs to consume before exercising, and completing blood sugar checks before, after, and during activity (Asif, 2014). Health care professionals have to build one on one therapeutic relationships with their patients by valuing their perspectives and understandings of diabetes as well as listening to patients' concerns about symptoms to address their unique needs of their patients.

Management

A collaborative healthcare approach is needed when helping patients manage diabetes. When working with patients closely, I have noticed that when a patient's concerns are acknowledged, listened to, and valued, the patient tends to understand diagnosis and treatment better. Compared to when there is a lack of patient-centred care, healthcare providers may opt for standard treatment rather than valuing perspective, which impacts the overall treatment and management of diabetes. When health care providers tend to follow standard treatment guidelines instead of listening to a patient's individualistic story and needs, patients become less likely to follow treatment and develop complications. Patients, caregivers, and families should be included in developing a suitable treatment plan with the healthcare provider to improve the quality of care.

It is also imperative to include diversity among healthcare workers with different skill sets, perspectives, and cultures in order to meet the needs of the diversity of patients we have in the hospitals/clinics/communities. A diverse workforce increases patient satisfaction and work efficiency while reducing healthcare costs. Health care workers who share similar lived experiences can build better trusting relationships with their patients through connection. Further, they can provide culturally safe treatments and exhibit a great deal of cultural competency to meet the patient's unique needs. Interestingly, patients are more receptive to the treatment when their experiences, thoughts, and beliefs are valued and respected. These patients showed improvement in their prognosis, had improved knowledge about diabetes, were able to cope better, and had an easier transition with making healthier lifestyle choices.

As a nurse, I have encountered several diabetes management strategies that benefit patients. Involving dieticians to develop meal plans for patients, including their favourite foods and restaurants, but also stay within the recommended dietary guidelines and portion sizes, so they do not feel restricted. Further, when discussing physical activity, it should be done in a fun rather than burdensome way. Involving fun activities and hobbies will help patients work on targeted weight but also help boost their mental health, improve mood and keep blood sugars in the targeted parameters. Involving family members in the treatment process is also essential in promoting active and healthy living. Many patients benefit from journaling their thoughts and feelings throughout the day, as it helps them vent, feel lighter, and to help them realize that the emotions they are feeling are valid and normal. T1DM patients are also encouraged to keep track of the food they eat to the best of their ability to assist with insulin administration. Many patients do not know the types of insulin and which ones they are on. They must be educated on their medications so when they are discharged, they are confident in their management of diabetes. Patients should be taught how to read food labels and made aware of the complications related to diabetes if not managed well. Overall, diabetic educators and nurse specialists are specially trained for this role and should continue to be expanded to meet the needs of the increasing population with diabetes.

The patient's family members also need to be educated on the specific diet that the patients need to be on, so they refrain from foods with higher carbohydrate levels. Family members also face reciprocal psychological impacts of the patient's diabetes diagnosis. Family members should be guided to the appropriate mental health services and therapy groups as needed. Health care professionals should be trauma-informed and able to build meaningful and trusting relationships with the patients, so patients feel comfortable being vulnerable about their diagnosis and open to asking questions. If a patient is not managing their diabetes, they should not be ashamed; instead, the healthcare provider should inquire about the patient's struggles and offer insights, advice, and support. Healthcare providers must focus on asking open-ended questions, are inclusive to their patient's families and caregivers in attendance, and provide digestible medical information (Ndjaboue et al., 2020). Once a patient is put on a treatment plan, they should have follow-up appointments to see how they manage their diabetes and if they have any issues or concerns. This will help providers adjust any treatment doses, prescribe further testing and provide any adjustments in their current treatment regime.

Future of Diabetes Management

Diabetes prevention and management remains a top priority within Canada. With an estimated 1.96 million people living with TD1M and a growing number of patients diagnosed with T2DM, research in the field of diabetes must continue. In Ontario alone, the cost per incident case of diabetes is $2930 in the first year following diagnosis (Bilandzic et al., 2017). There will be a tremendous increase in health outcomes if federal funding is increased for: mental health programming, medication research, access to diabetes clinical supplies, funding healthcare staff, and research for innovative technology. For instance, there should be programs in the community where diabetic participants can join and learn about diabetes, as well as patients can share their stories with other people and how they manage their diabetes or express their feelings on getting diagnosed with diabetes etc.Further, primary, secondary, and tertiary methods of prevention should be expanded; There should be refresher courses in the community which teach patients how to use insulin pens, take blood glucose levels, and education on how insulin pumps work. Moreover, education on signs and symptoms of diabetes, glycemic imbalances, and steps on how to treat these symptoms pre-hospital admission must be provided. It should also be noted the importance of telemedicine amid the pandemic and how effective and convenient it has become for HCPs to counsel patients. Lastly, understanding patient perspectives in managing diabetes is essential in improving health literacy and how healthcare providers can refine their care for patients and deliver health promotion activities (Adu et al., 2019).

As of 2022, with the COVID-19 pandemic and mandatory physical distancing restrictions, healthcare providers have geared towards telehealth to deliver care, answer questions, and support patients virtually. Digital health advancements such as virtual care should be assessed and expanded as they are an accessible means of care for patients needing medical consultations. Telemedicine is highly convenient for people with barriers to accessing clinics, hospitals, and healthcare facilities. Access to healthcare and the internet have increased concurrently; however, higher wait times persist. Overall, telehealth has been shown to reduce A1C levels, increase patients' satisfaction levels and the quality of their healthcare, reduce costs to get treatment, and improve patients' knowledge about their diagnosis (Ndjaboue et al., 2020).

Newer diabetic medications, insulins, and innovations to glucose sugar machines have been of significant help to T1 & T2 diabetics. I believe that in the coming years, with continued research and innovation, there is hope for better and more effective medications and insulins to help better glycemic control. In the past, many T1DM patients within the hospital setting have shared their frustrations with there being no availability of insulin infusion pumps. However, these pumps have now become a major part of the treatment and management of T1DM. Common among many patients I care for is the inconvenience of constantly checking blood sugar levels throughout the day. Research needs to be focused on assistive technologies and devices, which may include mobile applications that can automatically check blood sugar levels painlessly without patients having to poke their fingers. Such devices can also prevent hypo- and hyperglycemic episodes. Diabetes is one chronic condition that relies on patients' management techniques and factors that shape their disease outcomes. As listed above, factors like continued research in the awareness of health literacy, social determinants of health, and mental health are critical to improving patient health outcomes. Research on how mental health concerns can be improved in patients with diverse emotional experiences while managing their diabetes needs funding. The Canadian government needs to ensure everybody has easy access to healthcare and knows where and how to access the right resources and when to ask for help to seek diabetes treatment.

Key Points

- Nurses play a vital role in helping patients manage diabetes; thus, there is an increased need to staff more nurses in hospitals, primary care clinics, and communities. Nurses play various roles: being educators, providing clinical care to patients, helping patients cope better with their condition, offering mental health services, advocating for the patients and families, and making suggestions to the physicians and nurse practitioners as needed.

- HCPs and nurse practitioners should focus on each person holistically and understand their perspectives and symptoms pertinent to them while developing a treatment plan, rather than following standard guidelines of treatment for diabetes.

- Various barriers exist that prevent patients from managing their diabetes. These include unawareness of diabetes symptoms, lack of preventative measures in the community (i.e., primary prevention), financial restraints, belonging to underserved communities, living in remote areas, and lack of accessibility.

- Diversity in the healthcare team has been shown to help better patients diagnosed with diabetes. Professionals from different fields and religious and cultural backgrounds can build better therapeutic relationships with patients.

- Research needs to be catered towards specific sectors for better management of diabetes in the future, like mental health programs, mobile applications that can detect blood sugar levels painlessly, efficient medications, and more focus on telehealth.

REFERENCES

Adu, M., Malibu, U., Aduli, A., & Aduli, B. (2019) Enablers and barriers to effective diabetes self-management: A multi-national investigation. *National Library of medicine.* Retrieved July 5,2022. doi: 10.1371/journal.pone.0217771

Asif, M. (2014). The prevention and control of type-2 diabetes by changing lifestyle and dietary patterns. *National Library of Medicine.* Retrieved July 3, 2022. doi: 10.4103/2277-9531.127541

Bilandzic A., & Rosella, L. (2017). The cost of diabetes in Canada over 10 years: applying attributable health care costs to a diabetes incidence prediction model. *National Library of Medicine.* Retrieved July 6, 2022. 37(2): 49–53. doi: 10.24095/hpcdp.37.2.03

Clement, M., Filteau, P., Harvey, B., Jin, S., Laubscher, T., Mukerji, G., & Sherifali, D.(2018). *Organization of Diabetes Care.* Diabetes Canada Clinical Practice Guidelines for the Prevention and Management of Diabetes in Canada. Retrieved July 3, 2022. http://guidelines.diabetes.ca/cpg/chapter6

Kisling, L., Das, J., M. (2022). Prevention strategies. *National Library of medicine.* Retrieved July 4, 2022. https://www.ncbi.nlm.nih.gov/books/NBK537222/

Ndjaboue, R., Dansokha, S., Boudreault, B., Tremblay, M., Dogba, M., Price, R., Comber, A., Delgado, P., Drescher, O., Witteman, H., & McGavock, J. (2019). *Patients' perspectives on how to improve diabetes care and self-management: qualitative study.* BMJ Journals. Retrieved July 6, 2022. https://bmjopen.bmj.com/content/10/4/e032762

Nikitara, M., Constantinou, C., Andreou, E. & Diomidous, M.(2019). The Role of Nurses and the Facilitators and Barriers in Diabetes Care: A Mixed Methods Systematic Literature Review. *National Library of Medicine.* Retrieved July 2, 2022. https://www.ncbi.nlm.nih.gov/pmc/ articles/PMC6616628/

Pract, B. (2016). Barriers to effective management of type 2 diabetes in primary care: qualitative systematic review. *British Journal of General Medicine* .66(643), e114–e127. Retrieved July 1, 2022. https://www.ncbi. nlm.nih.gov/pmc/articles/PMC4723210/

RNAO. (2020). *Nurses have a key role to play in the prevention, treatment and management of diabetes.* Retrieved July 5, 2022. https://rnao.ca/ about/public-impact/diabetes

CHAPTER 8: AN INSIGHTFUL INTERVIEW WITH A TYPE 1 DIABETIC

by Gurleen Dhaliwal*, HBSc(c)

For those who live with type 1 and 2 diabetes, they are required to adapt and learn to manage to live with a chronic condition that can carry various complications and complexities. Managing diabetes is a life-long commitment that becomes a new normal in daily lives. Everyone's experience with diabetes drastically differs from person to person. Depending on the type of diabetes, age of onset, social support, access to health services and more, can impact how one manages to live a normal life with diabetes. I was interested in learning more about the experience of those affected by diabetes, and how we can use those experiences as a form of storytelling and empowerment. I aim to understand these experiences through a strengths-based approach that looks at diabetes from the perspective of not simply a condition that is rooted in stigma. My objective was to highlight the strengths of those who learn to live healthy lifestyles through the adaptation and management of diabetes in a way that works best for that individual.

This chapter highlights a completed 1:1 qualitative interview with a participant who self-identifies as 19-years-old, female and who has been clinically diagnosed with type 1 diabetes (T1D). I sought to gather their experience of living with diabetes. Various questions were asked of the participant and they consented to have their responses collected and included in this qualitative research study. Some of the main questions I was interested in included: What does a normal life look like for someone with diabetes? What does living with diabetes entail? Several factors affect how one manages diabetes, be it lifestyle or simply the weather. This interview moves past the surface of the disease and explores the depth of diabetes management.

How were you diagnosed with diabetes?

"I was in grade four around the age of nine. I actually remember the date–it was December 25, Christmas. The nurse who came in told me that 25 kids on the 25th of December were diagnosed with diabetes. So that was a small part of the day that stuck with me. It all started when I went on vacation. I was constantly fatigued and exhausted, which spurred my parents to take me to our family doctor. I did a urine test and he then told us that I had type 1 diabetes. The doctor kicked me out of the room to talk to my parents. While I was sitting in the uncomfortable waiting room chair, I remember feeling sucky. I knew what diabetes was because my dad has type 2 diabetes but it was still all unclear. It's been 10 years since and one of the things I remember quite vividly is really not wanting to deal with needles. I was admitted to the hospital immediately to help plan a regimen and understand how to adapt and alter my lifestyle. I spent at least a couple of weeks at the hospital and slowly adjusted to it all. I have to say, I did have a blast during the time I spent there. The arts and crafts room was full of construction paper that I would steal to take back to my room. We weren't allowed to take the papers out of the room so that's why I would sneak them out. My mom would also bring food from home (especially noodles because I was obsessed) which definitely beat the bland hospital food. All the nurses were super sweet which made the stay seem like a luxurious sleepover, or maybe that's what I imagined to not feel like I was in a hospital. Either way, it was a good time and that's all I could've asked for. I'm also eternally grateful for my parents because I don't think I would've had such a positive experience if they didn't instill such a positive mindset in me about it. They never made it feel like a burden or a tragedy that they were stuck in the hospital for weeks with me, or that they would have to worry about this life-long disease. We just took it one day at a time, and that mindset is still something I remind myself of every day."

What was the biggest lifestyle change that took place after your diagnosis?

"There weren't any major lifestyle changes that took place after the diagnosis. It was more of monitoring my diet and staying away from junk food in general. I was already an athletic child in elementary school and middle school. I was a part of the floor hockey team and the soccer team. So that activity carried through the years and it was a way I tried to stay healthy. I continued playing sports throughout middle school and the beginning of high school as well. I guess I also wouldn't really notice a huge lifestyle change even if there was one because our family already has one diabetic in the house. But overall, we were just more mindful of everything. I think one of the biggest things I underestimated was how much dealing with diabetes is a group effort. Even though I'm the one with diabetes, I rely on the people around me, sometimes even subconsciously, like my parents and friends. And I have to say I'm incredibly grateful for them."

How did you manage your diabetes in your youth? Did you experience any social hindrance?

"I was assigned a nurse as soon as I got out of the hospital. She was present at my elementary school and would help me with administering insulin. She would come during lunch hours and once I got the hang of the entire process, she would watch and observe to make sure I was doing everything correctly. The school was also very nice. I used to have lunch in the principal's room so I wouldn't be uncomfortable administering insulin in front of everyone. All the kids did hate needles. My close friends did know I had diabetes but it wasn't considered a big deal. My social life wasn't really impacted. I did everything I used to but at the same time, I didn't really know what having diabetes meant for me. I followed general guidelines as to when to put insulin on and what to be mindful of. My

parents were reluctant at times to send me out for sleepovers and events because they'd worry about how I was managing since I was young. Other than that, everything stayed the same."

How do you treat your diabetes?

"Checking your blood sugar is one of the most important steps. I used to prick my finger and put a drop of blood on a meter that reads the blood glucose level. Now, however, I use a sensor. It's a sticker with a needle attached to the end that I stick into my arm. There is an app I use on my phone that reads the blood glucose level. You could also use a meter but the app is more convenient for me since I have my phone with me pretty much all day. The sensor has to be switched about every two weeks. Based on your blood glucose level and whatever you are eating, you administer insulin."

"When I was younger and I would speak with dieticians, we would administer insulin based on carb counting. Carb counting is the process of counting the number of carbohydrates in your meal and using that to help you decide how much insulin you need. There's actually a lot of math involved. There's a correction factor which tells you how much 1 unit of insulin will decrease your sugar. For example, if your blood glucose level is 10.5 mmol/L and your correction factor is 2.5, then that means 2 units of insulin would decrease your blood sugar to 5.5 which is in the appropriate range. This example of course does not consider what you're eating, how much activity you're engaging in, be it walking or swimming, and your stress levels. When I was a kid, the range was 4-8 but once I passed the age of 18, that range changed to 4-10. This all varies from person to person. Gender, age, weight, and simply your individual body affects how you manage diabetes. I personally use needles to inject insulin however there are insulin pumps that you program that automatically administers insulin. They stay on your body for about two weeks until you change the

needle. You have to generally wait a year after your diagnosis to use an insulin pump. Because I used to play a lot of sports, I didn't want to use the insulin pump. As I mentioned, it stays on your body and I was afraid a soccer ball might hit it. It doesn't make much of a difference because a lot of diabetic athletes do use insulin pumps. It was just a personal preference of mine and an initial fear. The insulin pump is one of the most commonly used techniques to administer insulin."

What are some of the symptoms of high and low blood sugar you experience?

"Symptoms are unique to every person. Some people experience symptoms commonly known as high blood sugar symptoms during lows and vice versa. For me, when I am high I typically get very thirsty. Sometimes I experience nausea and a lack of hunger. When my blood sugar is very high for an extended period of time, I become really tired and sleepy. Lows are trickier to deal with because sometimes it takes me a while to recognize them. Most times, however, I know immediately. Commonly, I sweat a lot more during lows. The seasons also impact this. In summer, the heat makes you sweat naturally so this makes lows hard to recognize. It's similar to when you work out. When you sweat during that activity, it lowers your blood sugar. The same happens with seasonal heat. When the seasons change, it's harder to remember and consider the weather— especially living in Canada where winters are pretty long. Summer is the season I experience the most lows. When I have a really bad low, my hands start to shake and I get blurry spotted vision. Lows in general are easier to recognize because the symptoms are much more 'in your face'. In a day, I usually check my blood sugar about 6-7 times. With the sensor, it's easier to check it at my convenience. When I used to prick my finger, I'd check my blood sugar levels about 2-4 times."

How do you treat high and low blood sugar symptoms?

"Low blood sugar has to be treated immediately because the symptoms affect your brain and could make you go unconscious. The effects high blood sugar has on you are more long-term. Lows generally affect your brain whereas highs usually affect organs. I treat high blood sugar with insulin which lowers the blood sugar levels. If I'm not able to put on insulin, I walk or do some light exercise. For lows, I drink orange juice or mango juice to increase my blood sugar levels. I always keep a bottle of juice on me because it helps instantly compared to food, which is much slower. Also a fun fact: chocolate is one of the worst things to eat during a low because it's so slow in increasing blood sugar levels. It takes a lot of time."

How much would you say diabetes affected your life?

"Because diabetes has been a part of my life for so long, I don't really see how it has impacted my life in a positive or negative way. It's just normal for me. As my mom used to say, it's not a disease unless you make it out to be."

How would you say your eating habits vary from someone who is nondiabetic?

"I never skip meals but I do change the timing of my meals depending on my blood sugar level. For example, if my blood sugar is high before I eat a meal, I put on insulin and usually wait around five minutes to half an hour. The wait time depends on how high it is. Usually, my blood sugar goes low during 12-5 am and I eat snacks to accommodate it. I recently learned that this is because of the Dawn Phenomenon. Basically, when my body resets during that time, it uses hormones and a lot of blood sugar or glucose to do that. And that's the reason why levels

drop during dawn. For late-night snacks, I usually eat cereal or a piece of toast with strawberry jam. Ice cream is also a great snack."

www.ingramcontent.com/pod-product-compliance
Lightning Source LLC
Chambersburg PA
CBHW020708270326
41928CB00005B/333